LABOR RELATIONS IN HOSPITALS

Arthur D. Rutkowski, J.D.
Bamberger, Foreman, Oswald & Hahn
Evansville, Indiana

Barbara Lang Rutkowski, R.N., Ed.D.
Nurse Consultation Services
Evansville, Indiana

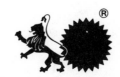

AN ASPEN PUBLICATION®
Aspen Systems Corporation
Rockville, Maryland
Royal Tunbridge Wells
1984

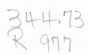

Library of Congress Cataloging in Publication Data

Rutkowski, Arthur D.
Labor relations in hospitals.

Includes bibliographical reference and index.
1. Trade-unions—Hospitals—Law and legislation—United
States. 2. Collective labor agreements—Hospitals—United
States. I. Rutkowski, Barbara Lang, 1945- II. Title.
KF3452.H6R87   1984   344.73′01881136211   83-22481
ISBN: 0-89443-582-5   347.3041881136211

Publisher: John Maroszan
Editorial Director: Darlene Como
Executive Managing Editor: Margot Raphael
Editorial Services: Scott Ballotin
Printing and Manufacturing: Debbie Collins

Copyright © 1984 by Aspen Systems Corporation

Library of Congress Catalog Card Number: 83-22481
ISBN: 0-89443-582-5

Printed in the United States of America

1   2   3   4   5

To our family

Stanley and Mary Rutkowski
Lt. Col. Donald and Hilda Lang
Laura, Michele, and Cheryl

Table of Contents

Preface

In *Labor Relations in Hospitals,* we have attempted to broaden the meaning of labor relations to include all of the major legal issues that managers in health care will encounter during the 1980s. In addition to current information about remaining union free and the various aspects of dealing with a union in an organized setting, the book provides the latest legal analysis of the newest concepts in equal opportunity issues, deunionization, OSHA compliance, wrongful discharge suits, collective bargaining, strikes, arbitration, comparable worth, reductions in force, employers' duties to accommodate religious beliefs, age discrimination, and other topics.

We have focused on cost-free ideas for implementing the "golden rule" and emphasizing the worth and individual contributions of each employee to the organization. Letters, checklists, and actual exhibits offer practical guidelines to hospital administrators for improving their organizational practices. A few examples include:

- tips to avoid wrongful discharge claims
- wrongful discharge and defamation complaints
- instructions for testifying as a witness
- anatomy of a union election campaign
- hospital letters in a union organizing campaign
- checklists for arbitration
- guidelines for the bargaining table
- police labor force guidelines during a strike
- what to do when an OSHA inspector arrives
- summary of steps for reductions in force
- what to do when a picket arrives
- activating a contingency force to operate during a strike
- legal no distribution/no solicitation and no access rules

- press release and letters to employees concerning the hiring of permanent replacements during a strike
- complaint procedures (communigrams) in a union free setting.

Barbara Lang Rutkowski
Arthur D. Rutkowski
March 1984

Acknowledgments

Arthur wishes to thank his parents, Stanley and Mary, for their encouragement and the invaluable background he received working in the steel mills prior to attending law school.

Barbara wishes to thank her parents, Lt. Col. Donald and Hilda Lang, for raising her as an Air Force dependent, which provided the opportunity to travel widely and meet people easily.

Both authors thank Tammy Welcher for typing the manuscript.

Part I

Pragmatic Labor Law

Chapter 1

Union Dynamics in Health Care

Future relations between employees and employers in health care institutions are not likely to be peaceful because of the many issues in health care over which management has little control. Managers can take steps to minimize the impact of unionization, however.

DEVELOPMENT OF A LABOR POLICY

Any effort to remain non-union requires managers to plan a total approach far in advance of any union threat. The labor policy for a hospital drafted by the board of directors should include measures that minimize the hospital's vulnerability to unionization. Four key points should be contained in this policy:

1. a resolution committing the administration to provide equitable treatment to all employees in their wages, benefits, hours, and conditions of employment
2. a resolution committing adequate funds and time to provide all managers with the information that they need to be effective in employee relations and knowledgeable in ways of avoiding unionization
3. a resolution committing administrators to the philosophy that each employee is important as an *individual* vital to the optimal functioning of the entire hospital team
4. a resolution expressing a commitment to oppose efforts of outside organizations to unionize employees

The board should make a strong commitment to resolve interprofessional conflicts among physicians' groups, nurses' groups, and other groups. Hospital practices regarding the selection of "supervisors" should be carefully examined;

decentralization of some administrative functions may be considered. The board and the administrators should examine the hospital's no solicitation-distribution policy, and the enforcement of the policy should be consistent. A mechanism may be established whereby the hospital can lend or receive assistance from other hospitals in the event of a strike in an organized facility.

MAJOR UNIONS IN HEALTH CARE

Hospital administrators must realize that the work force in full-time equivalent personnel in hospitals has increased from about 2,589,000 in 1970 to 3,280,000 in 1978. Of these employees, about 20 percent belong to a union. This percentage is remaining stable even though the work force in hospitals is growing by 5.5 percent annually. Furthermore, unions won 55 percent of all health care elections conducted in 1979.

While there are about thirty unions bargaining for health care workers, a few major groups predominate:

- The American Nurses' Association (ANA) and its affiliates have been bargaining for registered nurses since 1946. By 1980, the ANA represented some 105,000 nurses, more than any other union. The ANA and its state nurses' associations have been particularly active in California, Ohio, Washington, Minnesota, and New York; in a few other states, however, the ANA no longer seeks to represent registered nurses in union matters.

- The American Federation of Teachers (AFT), an AFL-CIO affiliate, began to organize registered nurses in 1978. While the union vowed to recruit 100,000 nurses in its newly formed Federation of Nurses and Health Professionals, it had recruited only 25,000 health care workers by 1980. The AFT boasts 550,000 members, who are primarily teachers; however, the AFT also represents a unit of physicians in New York City. In the 1980s, some experts predict an affiliation between the National Education Association and the ANA, both of which have a competitive relationship with the AFT; such an affiliation could weaken the AFT.

- District 1199, National Union of Hospital and Health Care Employees, is a member of the AFL-CIO and an affiliate of the Retail, Wholesale, and Department Store Union. While the majority of its membership is concentrated in New York City, District 1199 has mounted several aggressive campaigns in the Midwest and in the South. This union counts about 7,000 registered nurses among its 100,000 members.

- Service Employees International Union (SEIU), an affiliate of the AFL-CIO, has a total membership of 600,000; of these, 210,000 are health care workers. Some 20,000 members are registered nurses.

On June 6, 1981, the SEIU and District 1199 adopted a joint resolution to strengthen the bonds between them. This resolution is the first step in the joint efforts of these two unions to organize the seven million health care workers in the United States and Canada who remain unorganized.[1] The merger of these two powerful unions is likely to result in some 300,000 members in the health care field in the United States and some 40,000 to 50,000 in Canada. The headquarters for this merged union is Washington, D.C.

The SEIU also merged with a major group of women office workers to form an affiliate termed 925. The numbers stand for nine-to-five, focusing on the philosophy that working women need an organization of women, for women, that is operated by women. Its leaders, Karen Nussbaum and Jacquelynn Ruff, do not believe that District 925, an AFL-CIO affiliate, can replace women's organizations, but they do feel that it can attack problems of wages, benefits, hours, and working conditions. District 925 is the seventh largest affiliate of the AFL-CIO.

- Like the SEIU, the United Food and Commercial Workers represent service and maintenance workers as well as health care workers. This union, an AFL-CIO affiliate, also represents other health care workers and social workers. Since it began to focus on organizing nurses in the mid-1970s, it has organized some 700 nurses.

In addition to their direct work in organizing campaigns, these large unions are pressuring lawmakers to modify some of the existing legislation that allows management use of consultants during union organizing campaigns and legal deductions of expenses for professional consultants to avoid unionization. To understand the issue of management consultants, hospital managers should read "Pressures in Today's Workplace" to learn about the activities of management consultants, their proliferation since 1959, their methods and strategies, their role in a union organizing or decertification campaign, government subsidization, and issues relating to the Labor-Management Reporting and Disclosure Act of 1959.[2] Laws affecting the use of and activities of management consultants are also reviewed. Some authorities feel that management consultants should be required to make more reports on their exact activities; however, such modifications in the existing interpretations of the law would have negative effects for hospital administrators who need expert help in keeping their institutions union free.

ORGANIZATION OF PHYSICIANS

Organizing activity among medical students, interns, and residents dates back many years and was originally focused on the poor conditions and low compensation with which these individuals contended. The public probably first became aware of this activity in the 1970s when the Committee of Interns and Residents organized the first multihospital strike, which involved fifteen voluntary hospitals and six affiliated hospitals. The strike, which lasted only four days, was settled when the house staff's demands for more reasonable schedules, workloads, and responsibilities were met. This strike set off a flurry of activity in other parts of the United States. In 1975, the Joint Council of Interns and Residents struck three hospitals in Los Angeles, but these strikes were settled quickly. The striking trend extended to Chicago's Cook County Hospital, in which a job action for better working conditions and improved patient care resulted in an eighteen-day strike despite a restraining order.

This pattern of strikes and subsequent improvements was interrupted by the decision of the National Labor Relations Board (NLRB) in *Cedars-Sinai Medical Center*, 223 NLRB 251 (1976). In this case, the Board ruled that house staff members were students, not employees; thus, they were not covered under the National Labor Relations Act (NLRA). After recovering from dampened spirits, house staff in other voluntary hospitals began to organize anew. House staff in the public sector, unaffected by the *Cedars-Sinai* decision, gathered increasing momentum in organizing to obtain the best contracts possible. Because of the economic advantages of operating hospitals with house staff, administrators at five New York City hospitals had negotiated contracts with the Committee of Interns and Residents as of May, 1980.

Strikes in 1980 affected Puerto Rico, Boston, and San Francisco. On March 17, 1981, interns and residents in New York City struck nine hospitals for improvements in equipment, staffing, and better patient care standards. This strike lasted seven days at municipal hospitals and eight days at two private hospitals. The Physicians National Housestaff Association currently also represents some fourteen thousand physicians in labor agreements in New York, Chicago, and Los Angeles.[3]

PARTIAL ORGANIZATION

Many hospitals are in the unenviable position in which some of their employees, such as nursing assistants or licensed practical nurses, belong to unions, while other employees do not. One of the main problems of the employer in a partially organized facility is to avoid discriminating against either those involved or those uninvolved in union activity. It is unlawful under Section 8(a)(3) of the NLRA to distinguish between employees strictly on the basis of their union activities or lack of activities. While this provision seems simple enough, it can become complex during the implementation of normal management policies. For example, in *Solo Cup Co.*, 176 NLRB No. 823 (1969), the removal of union members from any profit-sharing plan because they have similar coverage under their collective bargaining agreement was held to be unlawful. In other situations, union activists who have participated in adversary encounters with management are often the first ones to be fired, asked to take days off without pay, or disciplined. In such cases, the NLRB utilizes the two-step test in *Wright Line,* 251 NLRB No. 1083 (1980), (1) to determine if the chief reason for an employee's discharge was the employee's union activity, and (2) the NLRB shifts the burden of proof to management to articulate a legitimate non-discriminatory reason for the discharge and to prove by a preponderance of the evidence that the employee would have been fired for the permissible reason even if he had not been involved in protected union activities. This NLRB rule for shifting the burden of proof in a mixed motive discharge case was upheld by the U.S. Supreme Court in *NLRB v. Transportation Management Corp.* (1983, U.S.) 103 S.Ct. 2469.

In *Americana Health Care Corporation,* 252 NLRB No. 57 (1980), an employee who engaged in union activity was dismissed after a patient filed a charge of abuse. The Board held such a discharge unlawful, since other employees with similar charges against them had not been disciplined until management had completed an investigation and so the evidence did not show that the employee would have been fired prior to management completing its investigation if the employee had not been involved in union activities.

Hospitals with no organized employees may encounter union problems when construction workers picket at hospital construction sites. In early cases of the mid-1970s, the NLRB interpreted Section 8(g) of the NLRA to prohibit such picketing. The Board modified its position, however, after several U. S. Courts of Appeals denied enforcement of the Board's orders and ruled that union members could picket as long as such picketing did not disrupt the operation of the health care facility and was not directed at any of its employees.[4]

THE AMERICAN NURSES' ASSOCIATION

The original purpose of the ANA was to "promote the usefulness and honor, the financial and other interest of the nursing profession."[5] Its purpose has changed little today. In contemporary language, it is to stimulate and promote "the professional development of nurses and advance their economic and general welfare."[6] A complete history of the ANA's Economic and General Welfare Program is available from the association.[7]

Professional vs. Union Activity

While the ANA began its work in 1934 when it campaigned for reduction of the workday to eight hours, its true role in collective bargaining began in 1944 when it determined that state nurses' organizations could participate in collective bargaining. By 1946, the ANA had adopted the Economic Security and General Welfare Program with its no-strike clause, but it was unable to force management to the bargaining table because nurses were excluded from coverage under the NLRA. In 1948, the ANA asked its state affiliates to refrain from engaging in joint economic security programs with hospital management to avoid accusations of company unionism. Even during the late 1940s, the ANA believed that professionalism and collective bargaining were compatible, although they restated their opposition to strikes in 1950. In the first twenty years, the ANA had made only minimal gains; while salaries had more than doubled in the twenty-year period, they were still woefully inadequate at an average of $5,000 plus.

The year 1966 was a turning point for the ANA. Its House of Delegates endorsed a nationwide salary goal of $6,500. Nurses in San Francisco and New York City achieved gains through concerted activity, and the state nurses' associations of California and Pennsylvania revoked their no-strike agreement. By 1968, the ANA had rescinded its no-strike policy in support of lawful action being taken by various state nurses' associations. In 1973, representatives of the ANA testified at congressional hearings in support of extending the Taft-Hartley Act to include health care facilities. When the health care amendments were added to the act in 1974, the ANA Board of Directors protected the association from charges of employer domination by excluding supervisors from Economic and General Welfare Program policy-making groups and refusing to allow them to play a role in the control of the ANA divisions' daily activities. The landmark decision in *Mercy Hospitals of Sacramento, Inc.*, 217 NLRB 765 (1975), gave registered nurses the right to be recognized as a separate bargaining unit.

By 1976, questions ran rampant through the ANA about the rights of certain nurse members. The ANA House of Delegates restated its belief that, because of the multipurpose nature of the ANA, directors of nursing should be included as members; however, the ANA Board of Directors began to study carefully its union activity and its relation to the other purposes of ANA. In 1977, there were more than 100,000 unionized registered nurses in state nurses' associations. The ANA also implemented a staff service program to help the state associations in hiring full-time staff members to carry on the union activities of the ANA in their states.

In 1978, the ANA targeted union activity as a prime priority of the state and national associations. It began to explain the nature of its union involvement to the members, many of whom had little understanding of the whole issue.[8-11] Even those nurses who did view the ANA as a union tended to see it as somehow different from other unions. Under the NLRA, however, unions are all the same and have the same powers. Differences in militancy among unions depend more on the personalities of those involved than anything else.

In "Open Letter to the Nurses of America," Barbara Nichols supported the union activities of the nurses' association.[12] She believed the question was not *if* nurses will be represented by a union, but *which* union they will choose to represent them. She considered the ANA the only reasonable choice. A flurry of other publications dealt with the dilemma of professionalism versus unionization.[13-20]

By 1980, the trend toward union activity in the ANA had gathered momentum. The Council of Local Unit Members was established through the Economic and General Welfare Program in response to the needs of local unit members, and funding for the program was increased. Not only did the ANA House of Delegates reaffirm their commitment to the nurses' associations as unions, but also the convention established a national strike fund. In 1981, the Board of Directors of the ANA made a bold statement that their number one priority is "to strengthen the association as a labor organization and to better relate this function to professional practice issues" at all levels.[21]

It is necessary to address the question of how a national professional organization can accredit practitioners, set standards, promote the nursing image, and provide both education and socialization among like professionals, while simultaneously functioning as a union. The professional side of the ANA activities are laudable; however, the problem created by its stated intent as a union is one of the biggest professional challenges of the 1980s.

1982 Convention

In an historic convention in Washington, D.C., the delegates of the fifty-third biennial convention changed the structure of the ANA from a trilevel model to a federation of state nurses' associations. Under this new structure, members belong to their state nurses' association, and the state associations are members of the ANA. The functions of the ANA in promoting legislation, setting standards, acting as an advocate for the profession, and protecting nurses' economic and general welfare remain the same. In the future, a national convention and a House of Delegates will continue to make decisions for the organization. Delegates will be elected by their respective states, one delegate for each 300 members at the state level. Dues will be prorated to the national organization according to the number of members in each state. Under this new structure, specialty areas and councils are termed societies, and membership at the national level requires state nurses' association membership. The economic and general welfare commission became one of five cabinets. The ANA House of Delegates will elect five members of the cabinets, while the Board of Directors will appoint two other members from nominees submitted by state and local units.

At the 1982 convention a very important new bylaw was adopted; it provides for ANA affiliation with other nursing organizations *only if the mission and purposes of said organizations are compatible with those of ANA, the administrative bodies governing those organizations are comprised of registered nurses, and those organizations designate the state nurses' association as their organizational representative.*[22] This forum, providing a liaison between the ANA and other nursing organizations, will meet at least annually to review issues affecting the nursing profession and to determine any collective organizational activity that should be taken in response to such issues. Details of this proposal as it relates to all areas, including labor relations, will be worked out between 1982 and the last biennial convention in 1984. After that date, conventions will be held on an annual basis.

The 1982 convention addressed many other issues. The delegates made a commitment to comparable worth and equal employment opportunity. They saluted nurses on strike and contributed to their strike funds. A majority of the delegates voted to approve a statement proposed by the Commission on Economic and General Welfare that discipline can be meted out to any ANA member who "participates or gives assistance to one or more directly competing labor organizations"[23] or performs activities that would interfere with the activity of the nurses' association in becoming or continuing as a collective bargaining agent for any group of employees. The group gave inadequate attention to the health and safety needs of nurses, however.[24]

In summary, the changes in the structure of the ANA and its constituents pose some serious questions to nurse-employees and nurse-managers who are not committed to the trend of the organization toward unionization. Nurse-managers, in particular, must make decisions about the nature of their personal and professional commitments. To determine how a typical local unit of the Economic and General Welfare Program works, all nurse-managers should read the ANA publication *Dynamics of a Local Unit.*[25]

IMPLICATIONS FOR MANAGEMENT

The entire issue of unionization poses serious questions for nurse-managers and other administrators. Should they belong to the state nurses' association and support the work of the ANA? What alternatives are there to unionization? What position should hospital and nursing administrators take?

Supervisors as Union Members

Section 14(a) of the NLRA states:

> Nothing herein shall prohibit any individual employed as a supervisor from becoming or remaining a member of a labor organization, but no employer subject to this Act shall be compelled to deem individuals defined herein as supervisors as employees for the purpose of the law, either national or local, relating to collective bargaining.

However, the union participation of nurse "supervisors" as defined in Section 2(11) of the NLRA raises some problems. Under the NLRA, a supervisor is defined as

> any individual having authority, in the interest of the employer, to hire, transfer, suspend, lay off, recall, promote, discharge, assign, reward, or discipline other employees, or responsibly direct them, or to adjust their grievances, or effectively to recommend such action, if in connection with the foregoing the exercise of such authority is of not merely routine or clerical nature, but requires the use of independent judgment.

The first problem is that union membership may place supervisors in the position of serving two masters, the union and the employer (see *Beasley v. Food Fair of North Carolina, Inc.,* 69LC ¶52,909,190 SE 2d 333 (N.C. 1972). Second, the employer has no duty to bargain with a supervisor who has joined a union. Moreover, a supervisor is not protected from termination for union activities as that individual is not deemed an employee under the NLRA. In discharging a supervisor who has been active in union affairs, however, the employer must be certain that such discharge is not construed by the NLRB as a violation of the Section 7 rights of protected employees (see *Puerto Rico Food Products Corp.,* 242 NLRB No. 126 [1979]).

Practically, supervisors, head nurses, and other department heads must make a commitment to management. Otherwise, they will be excluded from involvement in decisions that affect patient care in the hospital. Furthermore, because of union obligations, they may not be available to operate the hospital in the case of a strike.

Alternatives

Some say that the NLRA gives nurses a choice between banding together to have a voice in their affairs or losing control of nursing. They have danced around the fire by suggesting that nurse-managers should support the nurses' association union efforts and the professional unity even if it is to their personal and organizational disadvantage; that they should support the activities of the nurses' association that promote higher standards, credentialing, continuing education, and enlightened legislation and should simply ignore the union activities; that nurse-managers should welcome organizing activity, as it will give administration support for the things unobtainable otherwise; and that they avoid taking a stand against unionism, or so-called collective bargaining, because it will make their employees more determined and militant in their efforts to unionize.

In 1975, Richard Epstein spoke to the American Hospital Association administrators on "Labor Law: The Professional Hospital Employee." He spoke of the dilemma facing nurses and administrators in viewing the ANA. He said that individuals are placed in the position of choosing between two unsatisfactory alternatives. At that time, Epstein raised key points facing hospitals, such as the dues checkoff, membership encouragement, granting of support and release time to attend ANA functions, and free meeting facilities. He suggested that, since ANA was moving into the area of union activity, other unions might request similar privileges from these hospitals. Because many programs in the ANA are geared toward the betterment of nursing and health care services and because many nurses belong to the organization for those purposes alone, Epstein spoke of encouraging nurses to participate in events on a selective basis. However, he warned of the union-tainted nature of the ANA and of the problems of promoting membership. He empathized with nurse-managers who feel a sense of frustration about withdrawing from participation in the betterment of the nursing profession and concluded that the ANA should divide union and professional activities so that it is not a house divided.[26]

No better solutions are evident now. Most nurse-managers realize that they will have to make a decision about the ANA someday. For now, they participate on a tentative basis. Some administrators have asked them not to join the ANA, but in most places, it is still up to the discretion of the individuals.

There are many alternatives for nurses, but none is particularly feasible. Some talk of temporary collective action groups that form around a single issue; others suggest that nurses incorporate and contract their services to hospitals.

Managers often neglect one important point. Unions thrive only where management is arbitrary and unfair to its employees. Now is the time to take the needs, concerns, issues, and power of employees seriously. Managers should work in a positive manner to gain employees' input in the decision-making process.

NOTES

1. Bureau of National Affairs, "SEIU and RWDSU Unit Draft Plans for Joint Health Care Organizing Project," *Daily Labor Report III,* 10 June 1981: A-Z.

2. "Pressures in Today's Workplace." Hearings before the Subcommittee on Labor-Management Relations, Committee on Education and Labor, U.S. House of Representatives, 1980. Reported in *Daily Labor Report* 47, 11 March 1981: D-1-D-5.

3. Ira Michael Shepard and A. Edward Doudera, *Health Care Labor Law* (Ann Arbor, MI: AUPHA Press, 1981).

4. G. Roger King "Construction Picketing Notices to Health Care Institutions: The NLRB Alters Its Approach," *Medicolegal News* 9 (June 1981):15.

5. Publication EC-143 10M 11/81. Available from American Nurses' Association, 2420 Pershing Road, Kansas City, Mo 64108.

6. Ibid.

7. Ibid.

8. Barbara J. Brown, "Collective Bargaining," *Nursing Administration Quarterly* 6 (Winter 1982): 1–90.

9. Jacqulyn Gideon, "Unions: Choice and Mandate," *AORN Journal* 31 (June 1980): 1201–1207.

10. Ada Jacox, "Collective Action: The Basis for Professionalism," *Supervisor Nurse* 11 (September 1980): 22–26.

11. Barbara Nichols, "An Open Letter to the Nurses of America," *Journal of Nursing* 81 (1981): 1335.

12. Ibid.

13. Elaine E. Beletz, "Nurses Participation in Bargaining Units," *Nursing Management* 13 (October 1982): 48–58.

14. Gail E. Bond and Virginia Del Togno-Armanasco, "Public Law 93-360," *Nursing Management* 12 (November 1981): 27–30.

15. Gethsemane J. Campbell, "Is Bargaining Unprofessional for Nurses?" *AORN Journal* 31 (June 1980): 1288–1290.

16. Adrene G. Cohen, "Labor Relations in the Health Care Industry," *Hospital Topics 60* (November-December 1982): 33–39.

17. Lyndia Flanagan, *One Strong Voice* (Kansas City, American Nurses' Association, 1976).

18. Rachael Rotkovitch, "Do Labor Union Activities Decrease Professionalism?" *Supervisor Nurse* 11 (September 1980): 16–21.

19. Paula M. Stearns, "Making a Decision on Organizing," *AORN Journal* 31 (June 1980): 1208–1211.

20. Kathleen S. Tice, "The Director of Nursing and Collective Bargaining," *Supervisor Nurse* 11 (September 1980): 34–38.

21. Publication EC-129 10M 11/81. Available from American Nurses' Association, 2420 Pershing Road, Kansas City, MO 64108, p. 9.

22. "ANA Votes Federation," *American Journal of Nursing* 82 (August 1982): 1247–1258.

23. Ibid., p. 1248.

24. Ibid., p. 1255.

25. Publication EC-129 10M 11/81. Available from American Nurses' Association, 2420 Pershing Road, Kansas City, MO 64108.

26. Richard L. Epstein, "Labor Law: The Professional Employee" (Chicago: American Hospital Association, 1975). Audiocassette available from AHA, 840 N. Lake Shore Drive, Chicago IL 60611.

Chapter 2

The National Labor Relations Act

Enacted in 1935, the National Labor Relations Act (NLRA) was subsequently amended in 1947, 1959, and 1974. Since the 1974 amendments, the National Labor Relations Board (NLRB) has had the additional responsibility of applying the NLRA to private health care institutions, whether or not they are for-profit organizations. Health care institutions operated by federal, state, county, and city governments are not under the control of the act.[1] The 1974 amendments gave the NLRB jurisdiction over nursing homes, visiting nurses associations, and health care related facilities with gross revenues over $100,000 per year and over proprietary and not-for-profit hospitals with gross revenues over $250,000 per year.

Many subtle points and subprinciples of the law surround the NLRA. Case decisions are constantly modifying explicit interpretations of the NLRA. Hospitals with specific labor law concerns should retain qualified legal counsel to assess their situation in relation to current decisions and practices in NLRA implementation.[2,3] Furthermore, many other laws, both federal and state, affect employer-employee relationships:

- Employee Retirement Income Security Act
- Occupational Safety and Health Act
- Fair Labor Standards, Walsh-Healey, and Davis-Bacon Acts
- Title VII of the Civil Rights Act of 1964
- Rehabilitation Act of 1973
- Age Discrimination in Employment Act
- Veteran's Preference Act
- states' civil rights acts
- Tax Equity and Fiscal Responsibility Act of 1982 (TEFRA)

PURPOSE OF THE NLRA

The NLRA was enacted to eliminate industrial strife and establish the legal rights of employees, employers, and labor organizations. In essence, it protects the rights of employees to join or refrain from joining a union and/or to engage in or refrain from engaging in union activity. It clearly identifies the rights of employees to organize and bargain collectively through freely selected representatives. The selection method is a well-delineated procedure that may include a secret ballot election supervised by the NLRB. It prohibits unions or employers from interfering with the rights guaranteed to employees and specifies unfair labor practices. In addition, the NLRA delineates and protects the rights of employers, promotes collective bargaining, and eliminates some problems in labor disputes that affect commerce and the general welfare of the public.

RIGHTS OF EMPLOYEES

Section 7 of the NLRA gives employees much more extensive rights than many employees or employers realize:

> Employees shall have the right to self-organization, to form, join or assist labor organizations, to bargain collectively through representatives of their own choosing, and to engage in other concerted activities for the purpose of collective bargaining or other mutual aid or protection, and shall also have the right to refrain from any or all of such activities except to the extent that such right may be affected by an agreement requiring membership in a labor organization as a condition of employment as authorized in section 8(a)(3).

The phrase "engage in other concerted activities for the purpose of collective bargaining or other mutual aid or protection" has a broad meaning and can be applied to groups of employees who come to administrators to complain about wages, hours, or working conditions. Examples of rights guaranteed under Section 7 include the right to (a) engage in protected *concerted* (two or more) activity, even though no union is on the scene; (b) join a union, even if that union is not officially acknowledged by the employer; (c) participate in organizing the employees in one's workplace or in other organizations; and (d) walk off the job to secure better working conditions.

An example of employees engaging in protected concerted activity when no union is on the scene is *Dominican Sisters of Ontario, Inc. (Holy Rosary Hospital)*, 264 NLRB No. 158 (1982). In this case, the NLRB found that a hospital employer unlawfully discharged its emergency room nurses because they hired an attorney to express their objection to staffing patterns employed in the emergency room. The hospital claimed that this was an insubordinate action as the nurses had not followed the grievance procedures set out in the employees' handbook. The NLRB found that the nurses were engaged in protected concerted activity when they questioned whether the emergency department could safely function with one registered nurse on duty during the 11:00 P.M. to 7:00 A.M. shift. In hiring an attorney to protest the effect of inadequate staffing on patient care, the nurses were implicitly protesting their inability to carry out their duties due to the alleged understaffing—this was a protected concerted activity.

Union Shop

The NLRA permits the union and the employer to make a union security agreement under Section 8(a)(3). Under one form of such an agreement, new employees may be hired without regard to their union status, but they must join the union after thirty days to keep their jobs. In health care institutions, employees who have religious objections to dues and fees payment are exempt from such payments; however, they are often required to make alternative charitable donations.

Valid union security clauses are in effect when the following conditions are met:

1. The union must not be controlled or assisted by the employer.
2. The union security agreement must be in effect for the appropriate bargaining unit, wherein the union represents the majority of the employees.
3. The union's authority must not have been revoked in an NLRB-conducted election or restricted by right-to-work laws in certain states.
4. The union security clause must stipulate the grace period prior to mandatory membership. In the building and construction industry, for example, the typical union shop clause allows a grace period of seven days.

Representation of Employees

Section 9(a) of the NLRA provides for employee representatives that have been "designated or selected for the purposes of collective bargaining by the majority of the employees in a unit appropriate for such purposes" and further stipulates that these representatives "shall be the exclusive representatives of all the employees in such unit for the purposes of collective bargaining."

An employee unit is a group of two or more employees who are bonded by a community of interests and conditions sufficient for purposes of collective action. Not everyone can be included as an employee under the NLRA. Those excluded include agricultural laborers, independent contractors, supervisors, those in managerial positions, and those who have a confidential relationship with a labor relations nexus to management.

The determination of an appropriate unit is left to the discretion of the NLRB with the admonition that it must avoid "undue unit proliferation" in the health care industry. Section 9(b) of the NLRA states that the Board decides the matter for each representation case "in order to assure to employees the fullest freedom in exercising the rights guaranteed by this Act."

The appropriateness of a bargaining unit is decided on the basis of the "community of interests" of the involved employees. In other words, those who have shared commonalities in wages, hours, and working conditions are grouped in a unit. To make this decision, the Board examines three major factors: (1) the history of collective bargaining for the group, (2) the wishes and preferences of the involved employees, and (3) the existing organizational structure. The third point cannot be the determining factor in the decision of the Board. There is much debate between the NLRB and the courts of appeals about what is an appropriate bargaining unit in the health care industry.

Once the appropriate unit has been determined and an employee representative elected, that representative is the *exclusive* bargaining agent for all employees in the unit. As such, the representative must equally and fairly represent all employees in the unit, regardless of their activities or union membership. For example, in *St. John's Hospital and Health Center v. California Nurses' Association*, 264 NLRB No. 132, (1982), 1982–83 CCH NLRB ¶ 15, 270, a petition for an election was filed by the California Nurses' Association. The NLRB dismissed the petition because the association had a conflict of interest in representing nurses in collective bargaining while operating a nurse registry service, since the "customer" purpose that the California Nurses' Association had in its registry service was in direct conflict and competition with the hospital.

Section 9(a) provides that one or more employees can present grievances to the employer and have action taken on such grievances without the intervention of the employee representative if the adjustment is not inconsistent with the collective bargaining agreement and the representative was invited to be present at such a meeting.

COLLECTIVE BARGAINING

One of the major purposes of the NLRA is to provide a mechanism for collective bargaining. In Section 1 of the act this mechanism is made available

> by encouraging the practice and procedure of collective bargaining and by protecting the exercise by workers of full freedom of association, self-organization, and designation of representatives of their own choosing,

for the purpose of negotiating the terms and conditions of their employment or other mutual aid or protection.

In Section 8(d), it is stipulated that the employer and the employee representative meet at reasonable times for the purpose of negotiating in good faith. Upon request by one party, the other party in negotiations will commit any agreements to writing. During these sessions, the parties negotiate any and all demands over wages, hours, working conditions, and related matters. While the employer and the representative of the employees must bargain with each other to avoid an unfair labor practice charge, neither party is required to make concessions or agree to a proposal under Section 8(d) of the NLRA.

Some order is provided through Section 8(d) by its statement that a collective bargaining agreement stays in force until the party desiring a change in industries not involving health care institutions (whose notice provisions will be discussed later) complies with the following steps:

1. Sixty days before the contract ends, the party who wants to modify or terminate the contract must notify the other party in writing. If the expiration date of the contract is not specified, the party wanting a change or termination must serve a written notice to the other party ninety days before changes can occur.
2. The party who wants contractual changes or termination must meet and negotiate with the other party to reach an agreement on a new or revised contract.
3. If no agreement is reached, the party must notify the Federal Mediation and Conciliation Service and the mediation or conciliation agency in the state or territory of the dispute within thirty days.
4. The party wishing for the change or termination of the contract must comply with all terms of the contract, without resorting to a strike or lockout, for sixty days after the notice is served on the other party or until the contract expires, whichever is later.

If an employee strikes an employer during the notice period stipulated, that employee loses protected status as an employee under the NLRA.

UNFAIR LABOR PRACTICES

The NLRA prohibits specific unfair labor practices of both employers and unions. In summary, Section 8(a)(1), SPIT (spy, promise, interrogate, or threaten) states that employers may not

1. dominate or interfere with the formation or administration of a union, nor contribute financial or other support to it
2. discriminate against employees in hiring, retention, or conditions of employment as a means of encouraging or discouraging labor organization membership or activities
3. discriminate against an employee for filing charges with the NLRB or providing testimony under the act
4. refuse to bargain in good faith

Section 8(e), added to the NLRA in 1959, makes it illegal to write an agreement between the employer and the union wherein the employer agrees not to do business with a certain employer because that employer is designated as "unfair" by the union; this is the so-called hot cargo agreement.

Section 8(b) describes unfair labor practices in unions.

Section 8(g) prohibits a labor organization from engaging in a strike, picketing, or other concerted work refusal actions at health care institutions without first giving at least ten days' advance notice to the institution and to the Federal Mediation and Conciliation Service. This part of the NLRA has been upheld in cases such as *Service Employees, Local 200 (Eden Park)*, 263 NLRB No. 16, 111 LRRM 1613 (1982). In this case, it was ruled that a labor organization that did not represent the employees at a health care institution violated the NLRA as amended when, without giving the ten days' notice required in Section 8(g), its president and its business agent picketed the institution in sympathy with a second union that did represent employees at the institution and had given the required statutory notice before beginning its lawful strike.

ENFORCEMENT OF THE NLRA

The NLRA is administered by the NLRB, a quasi-judicial agency. The NLRB includes five members, who are appointed by the President and confirmed by the Senate and who serve staggered five-year terms; the General Counsel, who is also appointed by the President and confirmed by the Senate and who serves a four-year term; and staff. The offices of the NLRB are in Washington, D.C. The NLRB has established thirty-three regional and a number of other field offices in various cities in the United States and Puerto Rico under the direction of the General Counsel. Administrative law judges, who are independent of the Board, are appointed for life. Their function is to judge unfair labor practice hearings initiated by the regional offices.

While the NLRB can administer the NLRA, it cannot enforce its decisions and must seek the assistance of the court system to do so. The NLRB has two primary functions: (1) to determine an employee's representation status and (2) to resolve an alleged unfair labor practice. In sum, the NLRB decides who is included in a bargaining unit, monitors elections, certifies election results, and investigates and resolves any unfair labor practices that are in violation of the NLRA.

In representation cases, the authority of the NLRB is activated when a petition is filed. Following the receipt of a petition, Section 9 (c) (1) of the NLRA states that "the Board shall investigate such petition and if it has reasonable cause to believe that a question of representation affecting commerce exists shall provide for an appropriate hearing upon due notice." When there is a question of representation, the Board conducts an election by secret ballot and certifies the results.

A charge of an unfair labor practice may be filed by any individual, including an employee; the employer; or the union. The charging party must file the charge with the appropriate regional office and serve copies on each individual named in the charge. Such notice is usually made by registered mail with a return receipt requested.

Should the regional director issue a complaint, no further appeal is possible. When a regional director refuses to issue a complaint, the charging party may appeal that decision to the General Counsel, who has final authority in investigating charges and issuing complaints. There is no appeal of the General Counsel's decision.

The resolution of such a charge may be deferred by the Board, in which case it is handled through the grievance arbitration procedure of the employer and the union if certain safeguards and conditions are met. In deciding an unfair labor practice complaint, a hearing is conducted before the NLRB administrative law judge in accord with the rules and procedures that are applicable in U.S. District Courts. The administrative law judge and the general counsel have the power to gather, examine, and copy any relevant evidence; to call witnesses to testify; and to administer oaths and affirmations. They may also obtain a court order to compel individuals to comply with a subpoena and to supply testimony or evidence.

The findings of the judge and the involved parties may be appealed to the Board. If the Board determines that the charged party is guilty of the offense, it takes affirmative action to correct the inequities. It may authorize a cease and desist order, and it may seek remedies in the form of monetary awards or reinstatement of an employee with all privileges, including retroactive seniority. The Board may also order the union and the employer to bargain collectively upon request in order to reach a signed agreement.

Because it is both the investigator and the prosecutor, the Board sometimes loses sight of its neutral position. Hospital administrators who are involved in an NLRB investigation should consult their labor attorney to determine what relevant information or appropriate statements to issue. Careful planning of management strategies is imperative at the commencement of an NLRB investigation.

Theoretically, decisions of the NLRB are based on prior NLRB decisions and policies. Unfortunately, many NLRB decisions do not follow earlier decisions and policies, but instead reflect the political makeup of the NLRB at the time because Board members are presidential appointees. A task force sponsored by the U.S. Chamber of Commerce and composed of twenty prominent management attorneys analyzed hundreds of recent NLRB rulings and concluded that the NLRB's activist, antibusiness stance has damaged the Board's credibility and threatens the nation's well-being.[4] Not only has the Board sided with the union's position in many election campaign cases, but also it has unnecessarily interfered in labor-management collective bargaining relationships. The task force stated, "By involving itself in the collective bargaining process when individual employee rights are not at issue, the Board impedes the development of a mature collective bargaining relationship and artificially alters the relative power of the parties contrary to the regulatory scheme.[5]

Further hampering the Board's credibility and universal acceptance of its decisions is its unwaivering policy not to be guided by any decision of a circuit court of appeals. The Board has been rebuked by the courts in both the Third Circuit and in the Ninth Circuit for its decisions that registered nurses by themselves constitute an appropriate bargaining unit. In these circuits, the Board has continued to exclude other groups from such units, even though the courts have, in prior decisions, directed the Board to consider them in order to stay within the congressional mandate to prevent "undue proliferation" of bargaining units in the health care industry and even though Congress has expressed approval of the trend toward broader units in this area. In *In PPG Industries, Inc. v. NLRB*, 671 F.2d 817 (1982), the Fourth Circuit Court of Appeals severely criticized the Board for refusing to follow the Court of Appeals decision on the same issue in an earlier case:

> We acknowledge the deference due to the NLRB and its Hearing Officers when reviewing their credibility, determinations, and findings of fact. We cannot, however, defer to a legal determination which flouts our previous statements on the law covering whether a group of pro-union employees will be considered an agent of the Union. *It is the duty of the NLRB to apply the law of the Circuit.* (Emphasis added.)

In *Ithaca College v. NLRB*, 623 F.2d 224, 228–229 (1980), cert. denied, 449 U.S. 975, 101 S.Ct. 386, 66 L.Ed.2d 237 (1980) the Second Circuit Court of Appeals stated

> We do not expect the Board [or its hearing officers] or any other litigant to rejoice in all the opinions of this Court. When it disagrees in a particular case, it should seek review in the Supreme Court . . . absent reversal, *that decision is the law* which the Board [and its hearing officers] must follow.

(See also *Allegheny General Hospital v. NLRB*, 608 F.2d 965 (3d Cir. 1979).) The Board would undoubtedly receive more respect for its decisions if it would, itself, follow the decisions of the circuit courts of appeals unless the Board has appealed to the U.S. Supreme Court.

HEALTH CARE AND THE NLRA

The NLRA was amended in 1974 to extend coverage to private and not-for-profit hospitals. The NLRB had already exerted jurisdiction over proprietary hospitals with gross annual revenues exceeding $250,000 in *Butte Medical Properties*, 168 NLRB 52 (1967), rejecting the argument that such hospitals were not operating in interstate Commerce. The health care amendments of 1974 established formal notice and mediation procedures to minimize work interruptions related to health care institutions.

In the case of *Mid American Health Services*, 247 NLRB No. 109, 103 LRRM 1234 (1980), the NLRB found that the legislative history of the 1974 health care amendments to the NLRA, when coupled with enactment of other legislation specifically directed toward potential conflict between an employee's religious beliefs and collective bargaining responsibilities, establishes that Congress clearly intended the NLRA to apply to health care institutions operated by religious organizations.

Section 8(b)(7) of the NLRA establishes a time limit of 30 days for picketing when the purpose of such activity is to gain union recognition. While this section was not modified by the health care amendments, it is clear that, because of the nature of health care institutions, the picketing could be viewed as an "unusual circumstance" to justify a period of less than thirty days. The reason picketing at health care institutions would constitute an unusual circumstance is that picketing in and of itself could seriously impede the nature and ability of the hospital to treat critical illness.

In 1947, Congress passed the Labor Management Relations Act, 1947 (also known as the Taft-Hartley Act), amending the National Labor Relations Act, including the very significant amendment of Section 8(c) of the Act which is the so-called "free speech" proviso as it implements the First Amendment of the Constitution. This section protects employers' expressions of views, arguments, or opinions whether in written, printed, graphic, or visual form, shall not constitute, or be evidence of, an unfair labor practice, provided such expressions contain no threats of reprisal or force, or promises of benefit.

Section 8(d) clearly delineates the procedure for written notification of the other party in instances when one party wants to initiate, modify, or terminate a contract covering a health care institution. To modify or terminate an existing collective bargaining agreement, the moving party must give ninety days' notice (instead of the sixty-day notice for other industries) to the other party under Section 8(d)(1) of the National Labor Relations Act, as amended. Such stringent standards and notification periods are stipulated to avoid interruptions in patient care and to allow time for the parties involved to reach amicable agreements. Section 8(d) further requires involvement of the Federal Mediation and Conciliation Service as an additional resource in resolving any disputes.

Therefore, when either party wants to initiate a collective bargaining agreement or modify or terminate an existing collective bargaining agreement, such party must, in addition to the notice required under Section 8(d)(1), under Section 8(d)(3)(A) of the National Labor Relations Act, as amended, give a sixty-day notice of the existence of a dispute to the state and federal mediation agencies, in the case of a renewal contract, and under Section 8(d)(3)(B) of the National Labor Relations Act, as amended, give a thirty-day notice of the existence of a dispute to such agencies in the case of an initial agreement following certification or recognition of the union. To underscore the importance of this service, Section 213, Conciliation of Labor Disputes in the Health Care Industry, of the Labor Management Relations Act, 1947, was added to the NLRA. After the Federal Mediation and Conciliation Service has received notification of a dispute at a health care institution, only written notice from the union and the employer indicating that the dispute has been settled will stop the statutory proceedings.

Section 213 includes specifications that can be instituted to minimize disruption of health care services during a dispute. When the Federal Mediation and Conciliation Service is notified, it may set up an impartial board of inquiry within thirty days after the Section 8(d) notice was given to investigate the issues, make a written report to the parties on their findings, and make recommendations within fifteen days after the board was created, to maximize the opportunity for an equitable, peaceful, and speedy resolution of the dispute. Items that might be investigated by the board of inquiry are wages, hours, working conditions, training opportunities, benefit plans, promotional possibilities, equal opportunity factors, and other factors in relation to institutional size and resources, as well as community standards. Board of inquiry investigators also explore the settlement options that are least costly and most agreeable to all parties.

If the board of inquiry is created under Section 8(d)(3), it is in operation thirty days after the sixty-day notice to the Federal Mediation and Conciliation Service. If it is created under Section 8(d)(3)(B) in an initial contract, it becomes effective within ten days of the thirty-day notice to the Federal Mediation and Conciliation Service. Once the board of inquiry has been established, it has fifteen days to issue its report. Both parties are then required to maintain the status quo for fifteen days after the report is issued.

The Federal Mediation and Conciliation Service is not required to establish a board of inquiry, but once such a board is operational, involved parties are required to participate in it. They are not required to accept the recommendations of the board, however. The board of inquiry is intended to function simultaneously with the Federal Mediation and Conciliation Service. The primary goal of both groups is to avoid strikes or lockouts in health care institutions.[6]

There are two kinds of arbitration: *rights arbitration* refers to a dispute in the interpretation or application of an existing agreement; *interest arbitration* is the process of submitting unresolved collective bargaining issues to an arbitrator for settlement. While Section 213 does not show this discussion, the Congressional Conference Report strongly recommended the use of interest arbitration as a means of reaching a solution when there is an impasse in negotiations. In interest arbitration, the arbitrator decides the contractual issue and makes an agreement based upon the material presented by the union and management, as well as the findings of the board of inquiry. Like mediation, arbitration involves third party intervention on unsettled issues in collective bargaining. An arbitrator holds a hearing on the issues in dispute between the hospital and the union and makes a decision that is binding to both parties. Many experts point out that interest arbitration is particularly unsatisfactory to health care institutions because many arbitrators do not have any expertise in the health care field to decide the policies and procedures of such institutions. It is one thing for an arbitrator to interpret a collective bargaining agreement in deciding a dispute; it is quite another thing for the arbitrator to supply the policy to which both parties must agree. This is the reason that, in the private sector and with sophisticated health care bargaining relationships, there is very little interest arbitration.

Section 8(g) of the NLRA states:

> A labor organization before engaging in any strike, picketing, or other concerted refusal to work at any health-care institution shall, not less than ten days prior to such action, notify the institution in writing and the Federal Mediation & Conciliation Service of that intention, except that in the case of bargaining for an initial agreement following certification or recognition, the notice required by this subsection shall not be given until the expiration of the period specified in clause (B) of the last sentence of Section 8(d) of this Act. The notice shall state the date and time that such action will commence.

Through the years, the NLRB has been rather strict in its interpretation of strikes and picketing provisions. Not only are unions required to issue a ten-day notice, but also they are required to begin such activity within seventy-two hours of the time specified. If the labor organization does not start its action at the stated time, it must give twelve hours' notice before it does start. If such action falls outside of the seventy-two-hour limit to begin activity, a new ten-day notice must be issued. The purpose of such stipulations for health-care institutions is to provide them with the opportunity to make arrangements for the care of their patients during the strike or picketing. Management is not supposed to utilize this time period to "undermine the bargaining relationship that would otherwise exist," however.

LABOR-MANAGEMENT REPORTING AND DISCLOSURE ACT

The Labor-Management Reporting and Disclosure Act of 1959 places controls on labor unions and the relationships between unions and their members. Employers must report any payments or loans to officials or representatives of labor organizations, even those made only on a promissory basis. Employers should not pay nurses' dues or initiation fees to a union. Any monies paid to employees to influence the way they exercise their rights to organize and bargain collectively are illegal unless these payments are disclosed. Disclosures must also be made on labor relations consultants who engage in "persuader activities" and attempt to interfere with certain employee rights.

FAIR LABOR STANDARDS ACT

The Fair Labor Standards Act establishes minimum wages and maximum hours of employment. The employees of all public, charitable, and proprietary hospitals are covered by the provisions of this act. Bona fide executive, administrative, and professional employees are exempt from these wage and hour provisions, however. Hospitals may enter into agreements with employees to establish a work period of fourteen days, rather than the traditional work period of seven days. When the alternative plan is selected, hospitals need pay overtime only when the employee works in excess of eighty hours in a fourteen-day period. Under this agreed to plan, employees must receive one and one-half times their rate of pay when they work more than eight hours in one day.

NOTES

1. *FMCS Responsibility in the Health Care Industry* (Washington, DC: Federal Mediation and Conciliation Service, 1974).

2. Theophil C. Kammholz and Stanley R. Strauss, *Practice and Procedure Before the National Labor Relations Board,* 3d ed. (Philadelphia: American Law Institute—American Bar Association Committee on Continuing Professional Education, 1980).

3. Benjamin Taylor and Fred Witney, *Labor Relations Law,* 4th ed. (New York: Prentice-Hall, 1983).

4. Bureau of National Affairs, "Current Decisions of the NLRB—Troubling Developments for the Business Community." *Daily Labor Report* 243, 17 December 1982: A-1-E-1.

5. Ibid., p. A-1.

6. *FMCS Responsibility in the Health Care Industry.*

Chapter 3

The Organizational Campaign and Election

NO-SOLICITATION AND NO-DISTRIBUTION RULES

Hospitals that do not already have no-solicitation and no-distribution rules should promulgate them and post them on the bulletin board or disseminate them in some manner to all staff members. Those hospitals that do have such rules should immediately review them very carefully. National Labor Relations Board (NLRB) is in a state of flux because the Board's current five members have given different constructions and different rules in recent NLRB cases. Failure to secure a thoroughly competent attorney who specializes in labor law puts the health care institution at an extreme disadvantage.

It is extremely important to have *legal* no-solicitation and no-distribution rules if the hospital intends to take any action and possibly discipline an employee over a violation of such a rule. Of course, all employees must be made aware of the rule, and there can be no discriminatory enforcement of the prohibition, for example, against only union solicitation.

The general rule applied by the NLRB in solicitation cases, approved in *Republic Aviation Corp. v. NLRB,* 324 U.S. 793 (1954), is that a rule against employee solicitation during work time is presumptively valid, while a rule against employee solicitation during nonwork time is presumptively invalid. Nonwork time restrictions may be upheld only when the employer demonstrates special circumstances that make the rule necessary to maintain production or discipline. The Board has modified this general approach, however, with regard to hospitals, since health care institutions must accommodate the special needs of patients for a tranquil environment. Thus, the Board devised a special presumption for health care institutions in *St. John's Hospital and School of Nursing, Inc.,* 222 NLRB No. 150 (1976), enforcement granted in part and denied in part, 557 F.2d 1368 (10th Cir. 1977). This rule made a ban on solicitation during nonwork time presumptively invalid in all areas of a hospital other than "immediate patient care areas."

After receiving less than universal acceptance by the courts of appeals, the presumption came before the Supreme Court in *Beth Israel v. NLRB*, 437 U.S. 483 (1978). The opinion delivered by Justice William J. Brennan, Jr., upheld the Board's policy to require that, unless there is a substantial threat of harm to patients, solicitation and distribution be permitted in hospital areas where patient care is unlikely to be disrupted. The Court held this to be a permissible construction of the National Labor Relations Act (NLRA) as applied to the health care industry by the 1974 amendments.

In 1979, the Supreme Court had another opportunity to consider the Board's application of its presumption. In *NLRB v. Baptist Hospital, Inc.*, 422 U.S. 773 (1979), the hospital had prohibited solicitation by employees "in any area of the Hospital which is accessible to or utilized by the public." The Court held that a health care facility may lawfully prohibit all solicitation at all times in corridors and sitting rooms on patients' floors if such activity is "likely either to disrupt patient care or disturb patients." The hospital's contention that the rule was promulgated solely to protect patients and not to inhibit union activity unlawfully was supported by the fact that solicitation was permitted in such work areas as the nurses' stations and adjoining utility rooms. Although the Court held that the Board had ruled incorrectly when it said that the hospital may not prohibit solicitation in the corridors and sitting rooms that adjoined or were accessible to patients' rooms, operating rooms, and treatment rooms, however it held that the Board had properly ruled that the hospital had not overcome the presumption of invalidity as applied to the hospital's cafeteria, gift shop, and lobbies on the first floor of the hospital, which are used only infrequently by patients. The following guidelines were set forth as to which areas of a health care facility, in addition to immediate patient care areas, may properly be included in a no-solicitation rule. The Supreme Court stated that, "solicitation may disrupt patient care if it interferes with the health care activities of doctors, nurses, and staff, even though not conducted in the presence of patients."

The Supreme Court also questioned the validity of the NLRB's broad rule that solicitation may not be prohibited in public areas except for "immediate patient care areas." The Court explained:

> The experience to date raises serious doubts as to whether the Board's interpretation of its present . . . [policy] adequately takes into account the medical practice and methods of treatment incident to the delivery of patient-care services in a modern health care facility.

However, the Court refused to invalidate the Board's rule. Instead, it suggested that the Board review the "usefulness" of the rule itself.

In *Baylor University Medical Center,* 247 NLRB No. 178, 1980 CCH NLRB ¶ 16,752, the Board held that a medical center's broad no-solicitation and no-distribution rules prohibiting solicitation in all areas of the hospital, except in a few small locker rooms and outdoors on hospital grounds, unlawfully interfered with the rights of the employees to solicit in the medical center's cafeteria and vending machine areas, even though some patients and visitors used these areas. The Board noted that, for some employees, the vending areas were the only places they could gather during their fifteen-minute breaks, since the cafeteria was inconveniently located and had limited business hours. Furthermore, it was held that the medical center did not demonstrate that literature distribution in the vending areas would greatly increase litter or cause a safety hazard.

The Court of Appeals for the District of Columbia refused to enforce the Board's order in *Baylor University Medical Center v. NLRB,* 92 LC ¶ 12,961, holding that the evidence did not support the Board's finding that a rule against solicitation in the cafeteria was too broad. The court of appeals did not accept the Board's . conclusion that, because "attempting to contact 3800 employees located throughout various buildings . . . would be a herculean task," solicitation must be permitted in the smaller confines of the cafeteria. The court remanded for clear evidence to show that the task was indeed "herculean" and to refute the hospital's claims that the exterior grounds were actually more convenient for solicitation because of their frequent employee use. Furthermore, the court of appeals concluded that the Board did not consider whether soliciting in vending machine areas would cause disruption among patients and visitors and whether there were any alternate areas available for soliciting. The court indicated that a daytime ban might be permissible because of patient and visitor congestion in the areas, as well as the availability of the exterior grounds. A nighttime ban might not be permissible, however, as the cafeteria would be closed, patient and visitor congestion would be decreased, and the exterior grounds of the medical center would not be a feasible place to meet because of darkness. The administrators of health care facilities should be aware of the following cases on no-solicitation and no-distribution rules, particularly those dealing with no-access rules to off-duty employees:

- In *NLRB v. Presbyterian Medical Center* (10th Cir. 1978) 99 LRRM 3137, it was held that the NLRB lawfully found that the medical center had violated the NLRA by promulgating and enforcing a rule that denies off-duty employees access to hospital premises.
- In *Clear Lake Hospital,* 223 NLRB No. 1 (1976) 91 LRRM 1450, the NLRB found that a hospital unlawfully caused off-duty employees who were distributing union handbills at doctors' entrances to be removed from hospital premises. In the same case, however, the Board held that the employer lawfully erected no trespassing signs and did not violate the LMRA when it

caused an arrest of a nonemployee union organizer who admittedly trespassed on hospital property.

- In *St. Vincent Hospital,* 244 NLRB No. 71 (1979), the Board held that a hospital improperly maintained a no-access rule that prohibited off-duty employees from entering or remaining on hospital premises except as required by the work relationship.

- In *Eastern Maine Medical Center v. NLRB,* 658 F.2d 1 (1981), the Board found and the First Circuit Court of Appeals upheld the finding that the medical center violated the NLRA by promulgating and maintaining an overly broad no-access rule forbidding off-duty employees to be anywhere on hospital premises more than one-half hour before or after work, without making allowance for off-duty solicitation in nonworking areas. (See *Tri-County Medical Center, Inc.,* 222 NLRB 1089 [1976]). In *Woonsocket Health Centre,* 245 NLRB No. 80 (1979), the Board held that an employer operating a nursing home did not violate the NLRA despite an allegation that it promulgated a rule forbidding employees from returning to the nursing home after work hours, however. The Board held there was no evidence of disparate treatment or intention to limit the rule to union solicitation.

- In *TRW Building Div., A Division of TRW, Inc.,* 257 NLRB No. 47 (1981) 107 LRRM 1481, the Board held that rules prohibiting employees from engaging in solicitation during "work time" or "working time," without further clarification, are like rules prohibiting such activity during "working hours" and are presumptively invalid. The Board reasoned that there was no meaningful distinction between the terms *working hours* and *working time* when used in no-solicitation rules. Either term is reasonably susceptible to an interpretation by employees that they are prohibited from engaging in protected activity during periods of the workday when they properly are not performing their work tasks.

On the basis of these cases, a hospital is well-advised to follow the no-solicitation and no-distribution rules (long or short form) shown in Exhibits 3-1 and 3-2.

Solicitation includes distribution of written materials on the employer's property and the discussion of such materials with employees. Therefore, solicitation includes one employee's asking co-employees to sign union authorization cards.

There should not be disparate enforcement of the no-solicitation and no-distribution rules. However, although the NLRB has held that no one should be allowed to violate the solicitation and distribution rules, it allowed an exception for United Fund solicitations in *Hammary Manufacturing Corporation, A Div. of U.S. Industries,* 265 NLRB No. 7, 111 LRRM 1346 (1982). The Board reconsidered their 1981 decision in *Hammary* and held in an amended decision that an employer no-solicitation rule that made an exception for the United Way campaign but

Exhibit 3–1 No-Solicitation and No-Distribution Rule for Hospitals: Long
　　　　　　Form

Solicitation of patients or visitors by anyone on hospital property is strictly prohibited.
Solicitation, distribution of literature, or trespassing by nonemployees is prohibited on these
premises.

Unauthorized sales or solicitation of orders for any type of project or service to anyone on
hospital premises are prohibited.

Employee solicitation is prohibited at all times in immediate patient care areas, such as
operating rooms or patient rooms.

Solicitation of hospital employees by other employees or distribution of literature between
employees is prohibited during work time or in work areas, such as any patient care area. The
term *work time* excludes mealtime, scheduled breaks, personal clean-up time, time before and
after a shift, and any other period of time when employees are not expected to be performing
their work tasks. The term *work areas* excludes the cafeteria and coffee shop and includes
patient rooms; patient care floors; hallways; elevators; any area, such as laboratories, x-ray
rooms, treatment centers, or therapy rooms, where any type of service is being administered to
or on behalf of patients; and preoperation and postoperation preparation and recovery areas. The
term *work areas* includes any area of the hospital where persons visiting patients are likely to be
disturbed, such as corridors, sitting rooms that are adjoined or accessible to patient rooms, and
restrooms, but excludes lobbies and gift shops.

Employees are not permitted access to the interior of the facility during their off-duty hours,
except for areas open to the public at large.

---

prohibited union solicitation was valid. The Board noted that "the Board and the
courts consistently have held that an employer does not violate §8(a)(1) by
permitting a small number of isolated 'beneficent acts' as narrow exceptions to a
no-solicitation rule." The Board further held, however, that the facts as found in the
Board's original decision in *Hammary* indicated that the employer applied its no-
solicitation rule in a disparate manner against solicitation for the upholsterers'
union, since the company permitted employees during working time to sell

---

Exhibit 3–2 No-Solicitation and No-Distribution Rule for Hospitals: Short
　　　　　　Form

Solicitation is prohibited at all times in any patient care areas. In all other areas, solicitation
of an employee by another employee is prohibited while either person is on working time.
Working time is all time when an employee's duties require that he or she be engaged in work
tasks, but does not include an employee's own time, such as meal periods, scheduled breaks,
time before or after a shift, and personal clean-up time.

Employees are not permitted access to work areas during their off-duty hours.

---

numerous products, to conduct a raffle, and to collect for a flower fund, and itself sponsored the United Way campaign.

In a related case, *St. Vincent's Hospital,* 265 NLRB No. 6, 111 LRRM 1349 (1982), the Board stated that, although the Board has found that an employer's tolerance of isolated "beneficent solicitation" does not *by itself* constitute sufficient evidence of discriminatory enforcement, the Board "has never granted a blanket exemption to all charitable solicitation" and, in fact, has "consistently evaluated evidence of such solicitation in determining whether a rule has been discriminatorily enforced." In *St. Vincent's Hospital,* the employer permitted solicitation for sick employees, wedding invitations, housewarming parties, and the United Appeal on working time and in patient care areas. The Board found that the hospital's tolerance of widespread non-union solicitation constitutes substantial evidence of discrimination and a violation of section 8(a)(1) of the NLRA.

Another recent case illuminating the Board's reasoning involving disparate treatment is the case of *Holladay Park Hospital,* 262 NLRB No. 26 (1982). There the Board held that the hospital violated the LMRA, as amended, by prohibiting staff nurses from wearing yellow ribbons on their uniforms to indicate their support of the union's position during protracted bargaining talks. The Board stated that the disparate treatment was from the fact that the dress code was not used to prohibit other decorations on the nurses uniforms (i.e., Christmas pin), and the hospital gave no legitimate reasons that such enforcement of its dress code was for the welfare of its patients. The disparate treatment in *Holladay Park Hospital* and in the no-solicitation cases shows that the employer's real motivation is to thwart employees' concerted union activity. This is especially true if the hospital cannot show that the rule and its enforcement are necessary to the welfare of its patients.

The Board has also allowed other exceptions to disparate enforcement of the no-solicitation rule. In the case of *Lutheran Hospital of Milwaukee,* 224 NLRB No. 176 (1976), for example, the Board allowed a United Fund solicitation for a Woman's Auxiliary; in *Uniflite, Inc.,* 233 NLRB No. 159 (1977), it allowed solicitation for donations to the family of a deceased worker. However, it is recommended that such solicitation should be prohibited if the hospital wants to be able to enforce its no-solicitation rule.

EARLY WARNING SIGNS

Change is usually the catalyst that causes staff members to seek outside representation. Such a change could be the construction of a new physical facility requiring new support and work force patterns, the discharge of a very popular employee, or increased workloads due to a higher patient census or a reduction in staff. Dissatisfaction can result from the staff's need to adapt to these changes in the work environment. Some experts are worried that DRGs can cause such a change.

In the early phases of union activity, the professional organizer and a few key individuals who act as lieutenants in organizing the area of their responsibility keep a low profile while drumming up support for the union. There are many early warning signs that signal a union organizing effort is under way.

- Employee groups seem absorbed in conversation, but stop talking and disperse when the manager approaches.
- Formerly friendly employees seem cool and minimally responsive when the manager is around.
- Unlikely individuals are suddenly friendly and are frequently seen talking together.
- The type and number of complaints, even from formerly satisfied employees, increase. Hours, wages, and working conditions are often mentioned. Employees may speak to the manager more frequently in groups and send written petitions more often.
- "Outsiders" are observed on the premises, especially in places like the parking lot.
- With no apparent reason, the quality of work deteriorates; conversely, the quality of a poor employee's work improves.
- Employees are more frequently talking in groups before and after work.
- Patterns of early and late arrivals to work vary.
- Antihospital statements appear on the walls of the restroom and the cafeteria. Small groups of employees go to the restroom with different workers during the day.
- Loyal employees say that something is wrong.
- Grapevine sources seem to be drying up.
- Union literature appears in nonwork places.
- Legal terms start slipping into employees' vocabularies.
- A former employee who has quit or been fired periodically appears after work and buttonholes people in the parking lot or in local employee hangouts. (This person may be a union organizer.)
- During breaks or lunch, or before or after work, employees move around in small groups. (This is a time when union authorization cards are signed.)
- One or two employees representing a group air complaints in an aggressive manner.
- The rate of turnover either increases or decreases significantly.
- A previously popular employee is being needled. (This can happen when that employee refuses to sign a union authorization card.)

When the hospital is aware that a union campaign is under way and managers have been informed by loyal employees that union authorization cards are being signed, a union election petition is a very real possibility. At this stage of the campaign, employers should not overreact or panic, nor should they give in to the tendency to say nothing so that no credence is given to the rumors about a union on the scene. Staff members should be informed of the hospital's position on unions and of the important legal rights that they give up when they sign a union authorization card. The staff should be aware of the consequences of signing a union authorization card and of misrepresentations in the inducements of the organizer who asks them to sign such cards. A letter to the staff, as shown in Exhibit 3–3, is appropriate at this stage of the union campaign.

HOSPITAL'S APPROPRIATE UNIT

Of first importance in an election is to determine what groups should be included and who is eligible to vote in an appropriate unit. In *Mercy Hospitals of Sacramento, Inc.* 217 NLRB 765 (1975), the NLRB has found that registered nurses presumptively constituted an appropriate unit in health care institutions. However, in *St. Luke's Federation of Nurses and Health Professionals et al. v. Presbyterian/ St. Luke's Medical Center,* (CA-10), 91 LC ¶ 12,860, 653 F.2d 450 (1981) cert. dismissed (1982, U.S.) 103 S.Ct. 433, the court overruled the NLRB and held that such a presumption impermissibly shifted to the employer the burden of overcoming that presumption. The question (among other questions) of whether the NLRB's presumption that the bargaining unit restricted to registered nurses is appropriate was presented to the U.S. Supreme Court which dismissed the appeal, see (1982, U.S.), 103 S.Ct. 433.

The courts of appeals found that the NLRB *erred* in concluding that a unit restricted exclusively to registered nurses was appropriate in *NLRB v. St. Francis Hospital* (CA-9) 601 F.2d 404 (1979); and *St. Luke's Federation of Nurses and Health Professionals v. Presbyterian/St. Luke's Medical Center,* 653 F.2d 450 (1981). In addition, the Second Circuit Court of Appeals found in *Long Island Jewish-Hillside Medical Center v. NLRB,* 685 F.2d 29 (1982), that the NLRB's single facility presumption—that one physical unit constitutes a separate bargaining unit—is inapplicable to bargaining unit determinations in the health care industry under the 1974 health care amendments to the LMRA, 1947, and reversed an NLRB certification of a separate bargaining unit of 80 nurses employed at one of three facilities of the organizationally integrated medical center, which employed 630 nurses in all.

Other units and the cases in which they were found to be appropriate units by the NLRB are

1. Hospital interns and residents, in *Cedar-Sinai Medical Center,* 223 NLRB No. 57, reconsideration denied 224 NLRB No. 90, (1976)—residents,

Exhibit 3–3 First Letter on Hospital's Position Concerning Unions and Card Signing

---

Dear Staff:

    We have heard that there is some activity on behalf of a union to organize our registered nurses. We feel you should be aware of our position before you give up important legal rights by signing union authorization cards.

    This hospital absolutely supports you, its employees. We oppose union organization here simply because we feel a union cannot contribute to your professional development in any way, nor can it contribute to better health care for our patients. In fact, a union could take away the healthy exchange of ideas that we now have between the staff and management in providing a total health care approach for patients.

    We have and will continue to have good staff wages, benefits, and working conditions that are comparable to those of other hospitals in this area. You know that we have worked to establish the professional status of nursing, and you have the hospital's continuing commitment to the growth and development of nursing in the future.

    Why is the union interested in you? At one time, the nurses' associations were truly concerned about your professional growth and development. When in 1968 the American Nurses' Association withdrew its promise not to strike and started to organize health care institutions to collect dues for its economic wing, the association became a full-fledged union business. Most union constitutions that union members legally swear to uphold provide that a member must "continue to pay all dues, assessments and fines or other obligations of the union promptly when due in order to be and remain in good standing."

    A union representative may visit your home to pressure you to sign a union card. The union solicitor may make statements such as "Signing a union card is only to get an election." "You should sign because everybody else has signed." or "If you don't sign now, you may lose your job." Don't believe it! Signing a union card authorizes the union to represent you in all matters concerning your job security, the way in which you provide health care, and affects your own personal working conditions. Thus, it interferes with your ability as an individual to develop collaborative strategies and to participate in shared decision making that affects all nurses and their relationship with the nursing management group. Signing a union card is like signing a blank check—you don't know what it will cost you or what you are giving up as a professional member of our staff.

    If you are visited by a union salesman, please weigh what you are told very carefully. Insist that any union supporter supply you with facts. More importantly, if the union's facts are ambiguous or raise questions in your mind, please give management a chance to answer them and give you the straight facts.

                          Sincerely,

---

interns, and clinical fellows who comprise the house staff of a medical center are not "employees" covered by the Taft-Hartley Act, but primarily "students," according to the NLRB.

2. Physicians, in *Ohio Valley Hospital Assn.,* 230 NLRB No. 84 (1977)—the NLRB held that physicians as a class possess a separate and distinctive

community of interest apart from the other professional employees and constitute an appropriate bargaining unit.

3. Technical employees, in *Barnert Memorial Center,* 217 NLRB No. 132 (1975).
4. Business office clericals, in *Mercy Hospitals of Sacramento Inc.,* 217 NLRB No. 131 (1975), and *Sisters of St. Joseph,* 217 NLRB No. 135 (1975).
5. Service and maintenance employees, in *Newington Children's Hospital,* 217 NLRB No. 134 (1975), and *Allegheny General Hospital,* 230 NLRB No. 134 (1977). Further, the Fifth Circuit Court of Appeals in *Vicksburg Hospital v. NLRB,* 653 F.2d 1070 (1981), upheld the Board's finding that service, maintenance, and technical employees comprise an appropriate unit despite the hospital's contention that inclusion of technical employees, who are mostly licensed practical nurses, is inconsistent with prior NLRB rulings. However, the Third Circuit Court of Appeals reversed the NLRB's finding in *Allegheny* set out above that a maintenance department unit is appropriate in *Allegheny General Hospital v. NLRB,* 608 F.2d 965 (1979) holding that the NLRB's purported exercise of discretion was in direct conflict with its holding in *St. Vincent's Hospital v. NLRB,* 567 F.2d 588 (1977), where the Third Circuit reversed the NLRB and held that a separate maintenance department unit (in this case the hospital's boiler operators) is inappropriate in the health care industry.
6. Other professionals, in *Mercy Hospitals of Sacramento Inc.,* 217 NLRB No. 131 (1975).

In *St. Francis Hospital,* 265 NLRB No. 120 (1982), a sharply divided Board examined in detail the legislative history of the 1974 health care amendments to the NLRA and set forth new rules for determining appropriate bargaining units in the health care industry. In the *St. Francis Hospital* case, the Board found that a unit of only skilled maintenance employees is appropriate. Furthermore, the Board announced a two-tier test to be used in determining the appropriateness of the unit, starting with the premise that there are seven potentially appropriate units:

1. physicians
2. registered nurses
3. other professional employees
4. technical employees
5. business office clerical employees
6. service and maintenance employees
7. maintenance employees.

The Board then stated:

Accordingly, if a petitioner seeks to represent a unit comprised of one such potentially appropriate group, we then apply the various community-of-interest criteria to the particular employees involved to determine whether they in fact comprise an appropriate unit.

. . . While this approach may occasionally produce a case such as *Michael Reese Hospital and Medical Center,* 242 NLRB 322 (1979) where chauffeur-drivers were granted their own bargaining unit, we believe that such "additional unit" cases will be rare, and, in fact, greatly outnumbered by cases where separate representation for one of the seven potentially appropriate units will be found unwarranted. See *Mount Airy Psychiatric Center* 253 NLRB 1003 (1981) where we denied a request for a separate RN unit because of an insufficient showing of disparity of interest from other professional employees; *Kaiser Foundation Health Plan of Colorado and Permanent Services of Colorado, Inc.,* 230 NLRB 438 (1977), where we dismissed a petition for a unit on non-RN professionals because certain RNs should have been included; and *Appalachian Regional Hospitals, Inc.,* 233 NLRB 542 (1977), where we included business office clericals in a unit with all service, maintenance, and technical employees.

There was a strong rebuke from dissenting members Chairman John R. Van de Water and Member Robert P. Hunter. Van de Water declared, "No matter how many artful semantic rerationalizations of its health care unit determination policy that the Board may invent, it will not persuade the courts of appeals to join it in ignoring the express will of Congress." Chairman Van de Water then openly chastised the Board's failure to follow circuit court decisions:

The repeated refusal of the courts to uphold Board unit determinations made on a business-as-usual basis is sure testimony to that. . . . It is time for my colleagues in the majority to show their flexibility and pragmatism *and acquiesce in the process of bringing Board law in this area into line with congressional intent as interpreted by numerous courts of appeals.* (Emphasis added.)

Dissenting Member Hunter stated that the ruling is simply a "little more than a rehash of the same analysis that has been rejected by every circuit that has considered the issue."

Some important points can be gleaned from the landmark decision in *St. Francis Hospital.* Since the NLRB's explanation in *Allegheny General Hospital,* 239 NLRB No. 872 (1978), enforcement denied, 608 F.2d 965 (3d Cir. 1979), of how it determined that maintenance employees warranted their own bargaining unit was considered "imprecise," the Board again attempted in *St. Francis Hospital* to "outline the procedure we follow in determining the appropriateness of maintenance employee bargaining units in the health care field." The Board then stated that, in order to do this, it had been necessary for them to review the procedure used for other health care employee bargaining units, as "the analytical scheme in unit determinations necessarily encompasses all health care employees." The Board noted that, among health care professional employees, only registered nurses and physicians have regularly been granted separate bargaining units. The Board added that, although certain unique attributes generally distinguish registered nurses and physicians sufficiently from other health care professionals to warrant separate representation, they will not inevitably be entitled to their own bargaining units. In identifying the seven potentially appropriate classifications, the Board held that units smaller than these seven groups will not be allowed except under extraordinary circumstances. Finally, the Board stated that the restrictions they have placed in *St. Francis Hospital* on the number of potentially appropriate health care units meet the Board's statutory responsibility to prevent unwarranted fragmentation of bargaining units in the health care industry.

In order to maximize its chance of winning an NLRB election, it is natural for a hospital to want the largest unit possible to vote on unionization; the union has already established its support in the smaller units that it seeks to represent. It is especially tempting to push for a larger unit of registered nurses and licensed practical nurses or technical and maintenance employees. With the caution of avoiding "undue proliferation" of units, the hospital has a good chance of persuading the NLRB or the courts to approve the larger unit. However, would this unit be acceptable if the employees vote to unionize and the hospital must bargain with this unit? Some of the different employee groups may make unreasonable demands, such as compulsory unionism and excessive salary increases, whereas a smaller unit may make fewer and more reasonable demands. Also, the larger the group, the more jobs that must be covered in the event of a strike.

Although it may not be desirable to have service, maintenance, and technical employee groups included in the unit, a hospital should seek inclusion of management-oriented fringe groups, such as irregularly scheduled employees, and professional employees (e.g., medical technologists, occupational therapists, physical therapists, and social workers) to maximize its chances in winning the election.

SETTING THE ELECTION

A representation hearing is set to determine the appropriate unit and the date, time, and place of the secret ballot election. The NLRB and the union generally want the health care institution to consent to the unit as petitioned for by the union in order to avoid any substantial delay and to avoid the expense of an actual hearing. In the NLRB's haste to get both the health care institution and the union to agree on the appropriate unit, however, the NLRB may put pressure on the union to agree to include some "fringe groups" and part-time employees if an agreement has been reached on the date, time, and place of the election.

If the hospital attorney has postponed the representation hearing as long as possible and has waited until just before the hearing to agree to the unit, the hospital should have two months from the date the union filed the petition before the election is held. The election should be held on a Friday, if possible, since employers win more elections on a Friday. A Friday election allows the employer to make a twenty-fifth hour speech on Thursday. A Monday election gives the union the weekend to attempt to sabotage any speech made on Friday.

Once the details of the election have been agreed to, the hospital's attorney may formalize them by executing an Agreement for Consent Election. Under this agreement, the NLRB regional director has final authority on all questions relating to the election, including objections to the election and challenges of a voter's eligibility. In other words, the parties waive their appeal rights to the full NLRB in Washington with respect to these election items. It is safer to retain the rights of appeal and have the attorney sign a Stipulation for Certification upon Consent Election, which is the same as the Agreement for Consent Election except that it retains the rights of appeal to the full Board.

If no agreement on the unit or the election date can be reached, differences must be resolved at the representation hearing. It may be necessary to produce evidence to litigate the questions in dispute. At one time, employers conducted extensive litigation at the representation hearing over the appropriate unit in order to postpone, sometimes for many months, any election. The NLRB has changed its procedure, however, and litigation now seldom stops an election. Also, it is much easier for employers to judge the timing of their presentations and to schedule their campaign so that it peaks on election day when they agree on a specific date. Therefore, it is recommended that employers enter into a stipulation agreement if they are able to secure the most favorable unit and the election date they want.

The minute (literally) the election date is known, an announcement should be posted on the bulletin board (Exhibit 3–4). The union will attempt to notify the staff within the hour of the agreement (even if it is all accomplished over the telephone), and it is important for the staff to hear this all-important announcement from the employer. Therefore, the hospital's attorney should be instructed to inform the hospital as soon as he or she agrees to an election date, even tentatively in telephone conversations with the NLRB and the union, and it is relatively firm.

HOSPITAL STRATEGY

Emphasis on Issues

Many employers feel that the best approach to a union election is to take the offense and implement a hard-hitting, well-planned, and factual dissemination of

Exhibit 3–4 Notice of Election

As a courtesy to the National Labor Relations Board, your hospital has decided to allow an election to be held on hospital property and on hospital time. The election details are as follows:

Date:

Time:

Place:

This election is to allow you to determine if you really want to be represented by an outside organization that may be more interested in your money—in the form of dues of $12.00 to $15.00 per month, initiation fees, fines, and assessments—than in you.

We feel that our problems can be resolved without the interference of a third party and that a union would only make things more difficult for all of us. We feel that you may be required to surrender important legal rights to act as an individual, particularly those that you now have in the areas of shared decision making, in order to become a union member. A union steward may or may not want to satisfy you as an individual and may instead advocate what the group wants. Consequently, your individual concern may be sacrificed in the process.

Because we think it is so important, we are going to state the hospital's position in communications to you in the next few weeks. We will tell you why we feel a union is unnecessary and, in fact, why we feel a union could be harmful to all of us.

information concerning the real issues facing their staff. "Canned" campaign propaganda should never be used. All communications should be addressed directly to the issues facing the staff involved. At first it may appear that there are no real issues to be addressed. The employees must feel that there are real or at least imagined problems, however, or they would not have felt the need to seek out a third party.

Once it is clear that a union is on the scene, the hospital administrator, the nursing administrator, the personnel director, and the labor relations attorney should discuss strategy and initiate a planned, tactical effort to persuade the staff that a union is unnecessary. The first step is to take a stand, explaining why management feels a union is not needed and, if appropriate, why the union organizers lack insight into the staff's role in health care services. Management should take the initiative and always be *first* to advise the staff of any important developments during the organizational campaign.

Supervisor's Role in a Union Campaign

Employers must tell the supervisors of their employees what they can legally say while attempting to lawfully ask questions to secure information so that the employers have current data on which to act. Furthermore, supervisors are an employer's agents and can bind the employer in committing an unfair labor practice. Therefore, supervisors should be brought up-to-date immediately on what their role should be in the election campaign.

At this time, one person should be put in charge of the campaign. This individual should immediately contact the hospital's labor law attorney to review the information available at this time and to plan a meeting with all department heads, directors, and all other managerial employees who will be in contact with the employees being courted by the union. At this meeting, supervisors and department heads should be informed of the reasons that the hospital wishes to remain union-free. They should be given data to communicate to their subordinates and asked to report feedback. In addition, supervisors should be told to

- remind the staff that the hospital treats them as professionals and the union will interfere with their participation in management decisions that will affect their entire careers
- inform the staff that the hospital prefers to deal with them directly, rather than through a union that does not understand patient care problems
- inform the staff of the disadvantages of belonging to a union such as *strikes, picket line duty, monthly union dues,* and *strike assessments, even for strikes at other hospitals*
- remind the staff that the hospital has always tried to allow them the fullest professional development by supporting seminars, workshops, and other programs and by encouraging them to have a voice in their affairs
- inform the staff about the benefits they presently enjoy and compare their wages and benefits with those of unionized concerns that offer lower and less desirable benefits
- inform the staff that they may be cooperating with a few militant staff members who want power for themselves
- inform the staff that the union cannot prevent layoffs and discharges, nor can it guarantee that employees will not be required to work on weekends and holidays nor can it guarantee any certain scheduling arrangement
- inform the staff that the union's only weapon is to call a strike and during a strike they not only do not have wages, but also lose their health insurance and, in most states, do not receive unemployment compensation
- inform the staff that they may lose their jobs in the event of an economic strike because the law permits the hospital to hire a permanent replacement for anyone who engages in such a strike
- inform the staff that no union can make a hospital agree to anything it does not wish to, or pay any more than it is willing or able to do
- inform the staff that a union card says they accept membership—not an election—and that they may have a union without a vote
- inform the staff of any untrue or misleading statements made by an organizer, handbills, or any medium of union propaganda and provide the staff with the correct facts

- inform the staff that the hospital opposes the principle of compulsory union membership
- inform the staff that patients will never understand their withholding care in a strike and ask if they are willing to make such a serious decision affecting their patients
- keep outside organizers out of patient care areas when they are organizing
- ask staff member if they saw the hospital's latest communique and if they have any questions on it
- make or enforce any rules requiring that solicitation of membership or discussion of union affairs be conducted outside of work time. (Remember, however, that an employee may solicit and discuss unionism at breaks, lunch, and before or after a shift, even on hospital premises, only if it does not disrupt other workers during their work time. The staff may never solicit and discuss unionism in patient care areas.)
- lay off, discipline, and discharge for cause, so long as such action follows customary practice and is done without regard to an employee's union activity
- make assignments of preferred work, overtime, and shift without reference to an employee's participation or nonparticipation in union activities
- enforce the hospital's rules impartially and in accordance with customary action, irrespective of the employee's activity in a union

Inasmuch as the supervisors are going to be responsible for communicating with those employees in their departments, they should be shown all campaign propaganda before it is transmitted to the staff. For example, a list of the most important and common disadvantages of a union may be given to the staff (Exhibit 3–5).

It is also necessary to review with all the supervisors and department heads what they cannot say and do. The easiest way to remember the broad general principles is to use the acronym SPIT:

1. Do not *s*py on employee union activities.
2. Do not *p*romise employees anything that revolves around union activity or lack of union activity.
3. Do not *i*nterrogate employees about union activities
4. Do not *t*hreaten employees because of their union involvement.

If, in addition, supervisors do not ask whether employees have signed a union card or whether they are for or against the union, they will have, in most cases, stayed within the boundaries of the law.

More specifically, supervisors must not:

- threaten or actually discharge, discipline, transfer, or lay off employees because of their activities on behalf of the union

Exhibit 3–5 Disadvantages of a Union to Employees

1. **Strikes**. Strikers may lose wages, insurance, and even jobs (when the hospital continues operations and hires permanent replacements). Patient care may become inadequate because of the strike.
2. **Red Tape**. Time and money must be spent by employees, union stewards, and hospital supervisors in costly arbitration of grievances that are often groundless, filed for political purposes, or filed for the benefit of the union.
3. **Dues, initiation fees**. There is additional expense to the employees, who do not have to pay dues to keep their jobs now, and to management, for payroll deduction of dues is costly and time-consuming.
4. **Increased cost**. Collective bargaining negotiations over weeks and months, time spent in the grievance procedure, job shrinkage (i.e., unions want more employees doing less work or the old case of an electrician being the only one to turn on the light switch), attorney fees, management time away from their usual job responsibilities, and, if excessive union demands are met, higher production costs are associated with unions. A conservative estimate is that any union will cost a hospital an additional 25 percent in operating costs without any increase in efficiency.
5. **Discipline policies**. The hospital's discipline policies, as well as its promotional decisions, are always questioned by the union. A union may seriously impair a hospital's right to exercise all of its ordinary management prerogatives.
6. **Seniority**. Becomes the "great leveler". Unions do not want individual merit to be awarded either in promotions or in merit increases. In representing all employees they politically can't say one employee is better and thus more deserving than another employee.
7. **Decrease in employee initiative.** Alert employees may be overlooked in favor of union employees who are union officials.
8. **Rigid classification of jobs**. The second biggest waste and expense that unionism can bring a hospital is to narrow employees' work assignments.
9. **Union fines.** Employee morale may decrease because of union fines.
10. **Deterioration of employee-management relations**. Friendly and individual relations between employees and management concerning the handling of complaints and changing of working conditions may cease.
11. **Climate of mistrust**. Because it is much easier to justify a union to dissatisfied and unhappy employees, union professionals must magnify grievances and create a mistrust of management in employees.
12. **Loss of employee freedom**. When a union comes in, employees lose their freedom to handle their own problems individually and directly with management.
13. **Loss of real job security**. Steady operations without interruptions due to strikes and picket lines keep the hospital's business successful so that employees have real job security.
14. **Loss of employees' right to think, work, and act as individuals**. Once a union is voted in, it can use threats, ridicule, misrepresentation, and browbeating to make work disagreeable for employees who do not conform to the ideas of the union leaders.

- threaten that the hospital will close or drastically reduce operations if employees choose to join a union
- discriminate against employees who are actively supporting the union by intentionally assigning undesirable work to them
- discipline or penalize employees who are actively supporting a union for an infraction that non-union employees are permitted to commit without being disciplined
- insist that staff members talk about the union if they do not want to discuss it
- make any work assignment for the purpose of causing an employee who has been active on behalf of the union to resign
- tell employees that they will be discharged or disciplined if they are active on behalf of the union
- visit the homes of employees for the purpose of urging them to reject the union
- ask employees if they have signed a union authorization card or if they have attended any union meetings

Although supervisors cannot interrogate employees, they can obtain information by talking daily with them. It is perfectly legal to start an interview as follows:

- "How are things going?"
- "Did you see the latest communique from the hospital (or the union, if such is the case)? What did you think?"
- "Mary, I think a lot of you and your opinions, and I would like to talk to you frankly about this union situation. Do you have any objections to discussing it? Do you have any questions about what the union can and cannot do for you?"
- "Do you have any questions concerning any of the rumors about the union?"
- "I frankly don't see how the union could help the staff or help in the decisions affecting nursing care."

If a staff member in any way feels uncomfortable in talking to a supervisor about the union, the supervisor should immediately end the conversation by assuring the employee that (a) all employees have the right to be for or against the union, (b) an employee's stand for or against the union will have no bearing on that employee's position with the hospital, and (c) the hospital intends to run a completely legal campaign.

In concluding an interview with an employee, the supervisor should write down any questions that he or she has not been able to answer directly. An employee must always feel that management will provide any information it can lawfully disseminate. Thus, the supervisor should never allow a question to go unanswered simply because there may be some legal problems with answering the question. The appropriate answer should be secured and immediately given to the employee. The supervisor should make it clear to the employee that he or she is personally 100 percent against the union. Finally, the supervisor might ask for the employee's help in the upcoming election for the benefit of all the employees, their families, the patients, and the hospital.

NEED TO KNOW THE OPPONENT

In *Sierra Vista Hospital, Inc., and California Nurses' Association, affiliated with the American Nurses' Association,* 241 NLRB No. 107, 1978-79 CCH NLRB ¶15,685, the NLRB said about the California and all other state nurses' associations:

> At the outset, therefore, we stress that "labor organization" status under the Act bears no relation to a delegation and/or local control of bargaining, and we disavow any implication to the contrary in prior Board decisions involving nurses' associations. As long as nurse-employees participate in the association and one of its purposes is representing employees in collective bargaining, *a nurses' association,* like any other, meets the definition of "labor organization" in Section 2(5) of the Act.

Nurses who have sought out a state nurses' association and then claim that the association is not a union but merely a professional association are setting up a smoke screen, according to the NLRB finding. Furthermore, the mere fact that the nurses' association can strike, stopping the delivery of patient care, shows that they are a union.

Information about a Particular Union

The hospital must gather all the data it can about the union that is organizing it; the union has undoubtedly gathered as much information as possible about the hospital. Knowledge of the adversary is necessary in any election campaign. The first step is to determine the official complete name of the union, including the local number if there is one, since unions must file reports with the U.S. Department of Labor. The exact name of the union and its reporting number can be obtained from the Register of Reporting Labor Organizations, published by the Labor Management Services Administration, U.S. Department of Labor.

The Labor Organization Information Report (LM-1 report) contains the union's officers, its fees, and dues, as well as certain parts of its constitution and bylaws, provisions on levying of assessments, selection of stewards, and strike authorization procedures. The Labor Organization Annual Report (LM-2 report) is a yearly financial report that gives not only the salaries of the union's officials but, more importantly, the salary of the representative who is attempting to organize the staff. It also includes the administrative expense of maintaining the union, which can be used to determine what portion of the members' dues goes into the union's coffers. This report also gives the amount of the union's strike fund and disbursements to its members as strike benefits.

These reports can be obtained from the Disclosure Bureau, Labor Management Services Administration.[1] The union's constitution and bylaws are available from the Office of Labor-Management and Welfare-Pension Reports.[2] A listing of the union's strikes by year and by state may be obtained from the Bureau of National Affairs, Inc.,[3] for a reasonable fee per year of search. For a modest fee, this organization will also send the union's latest LM-1 report, their LM-2 report, and their constitution and bylaws. Requesting these documents through the Bureau of National Affairs rather than the Department of Labor may eliminate delay in securing them. They also have union contracts that may prove helpful. Finally, newspaper clippings of a union's strikes over a period of years can be obtained from the state Chamber of Commerce, labor relations department, or the state hospital association.

With these documents in hand, the hospital can factually and dramatically describe the pitfalls of unionization:

- Under its constitution and bylaws, the union has the legal power to require members to pay initiation fees and dues, as well as to charge them strike assessments for strikes at other hospitals.
- A union can fine its members for conduct unbecoming a union member or for some other vague violation of union rules and may go to court to make them pay those fines.
- The union can also fine its members for crossing a picket line to provide critical and necessary health care services to patients during any work stoppage. These obligations to the union can total hundreds and even thousands of dollars.
- The union spends most of its budget on salaries and administrative expenses for the union coffers.
- The union can call its members out on strike in most cases without a secret ballot vote. In many cases, only a majority of those *present* at a union meeting vote to strike. In other words, if only 60 people of a bargaining unit of 200 attend a union meeting, those 60 people decide if there will be a strike.
- In most cases, strike benefits are earned by taking picket duty and average about twenty-five dollars per week. Furthermore, the union has only limited funds for strike benefits.

- In many cases, the union does not obtain a contract, even after many months of negotiations.

Showing of Interest

The union must have a 30 percent showing of interest before the NLRB will process its election petition. This is a discretionary standard imposed by the Board. The hospital can request that the regional office check the showing of interest against a list of employees that it supplies and their signatures against employees' W-4 forms. Rarely will the Board refuse to process the election petition.

There is no reason to give out the names of the staff at this time. The hospital is required to supply the names and addresses of its staff when they are formally requested by the NLRB regional director, however. This is referred to as the Excelsior list, referring to the Board's decision in *Excelsior Underwear, Inc.,* 156 NLRB 1236 (1966), that employers must furnish the Board with a list of all the names and addresses of the staff in the unit covered; the Board, in turn, furnishes the list to the union. The Excelsior list must be furnished within seven days after the regional director's decision directing an election or within seven days after a consent agreement is approved.

NLRB NOTICES

When forwarding the election petition to the employer, the NLRB also forwards an NLRB notice allegedly calling the staff's attention to their rights under the NLRA. A quick review of this notice shows that it emphasizes what the employer cannot do, thus implying that the NLRB is in favor of union organization. This announcement should not be posted. The hospital should not confuse this announcement with the actual notice of the election that establishes the date, time, and polling place and has a sample ballot inscribed on it. The election notice comes seven to ten days before the election and must be posted within seventy-two hours of the election. Failure to post this notice is grounds for setting aside the election.

ACTUAL CAMPAIGN FOR REGISTERED NURSES

In a small town in Kentucky, a nurse who had been discharged by a health care institution for negligent patient care instigated a walkout by the hospital's thirty-two registered nurses. She then set up small group meetings among the nurses to discuss, not unionization, but broad general issues of hospital policies on patient care and nursing practices. She then invited everyone to attend a general meeting to discuss nursing working conditions and patient care, requesting nurses to band together to use their skill and knowledge to benefit the profession, to improve patient care, and to get her job back.

After a few weeks, more formal communications were forwarded to all the nurses on union letterhead. During this preliminary stage of the campaign, the union was acting sub rosa. Meetings were usually held with a select few employees, prompted by the terminated nurse, either at homes or restaurants. At this point, the union organizer was trying to

1. solidify support among those who had been in recent contact through the small group meetings
2. build new support through inside leadership in the hospital
3. secure a list of employee names and addresses
4. obtain a list of managers and supervisors who were considered unfair
5. compile a litany of "wrongs" or complaints to add to the discharge, such as scheduling; lack of job security; sex discrimination, particularly in pay; physician abuse; sexual harassment; and failure to heed complaints

Any organizer maintains a record of complaints, classifying them as individual, floorwide, or institutionwide, and is very interested in the hospital's methods of handling complaints, layoff policies, and recent discharges. In this particular campaign, the prime target was the claimed arbitrary discharge of the registered nurse.

The hospital's campaign strategy proved to be extremely effective. The common thread throughout the hospital's campaign was that it had shown its fairness in dealing with all its nurses. It not only showed that the discharge of the nurse was justified, but also established channels of communication to answer all questions and to explain to the registered nurses why it felt unionization would be detrimental to their professional growth and development. In its campaign, the hospital took the following steps:

1. The hospital, while not overreacting, took the offensive and pointed out that the discharged member of the staff was doing all the complaining—for obvious reasons. The many contributions the hospital had made to the professional development of its nursing staff, as well as in the areas of wages and fringe benefits were noted.
2. The hospital administrator held weekly breakfast meetings with the nurses to discuss issues relating to the election campaign and stated the hospital's position on such issues. Any questions that could not be answered immediately were followed up and a response given as soon as possible.
3. The fact that participatory management and the staff's involvement affecting patient care was stressed. The hospital brought out that its registered nurses

were self-actualized through a multidisciplinary team approach and that in the hospital's view, bringing in outsiders would interfere in this relationship. The hospital pointed out that with a union being the exclusive representative over wages, hours, and working conditions (particularly as those conditions affected patient care), this exclusiveness would undermine the ability of the nursing staff to share in decision making with the nursing management group.

4. An in-house committee was established by the nurses themselves to correct any misstatements made by the union or other nurses. Some misrepresentations were corrected by letters written from the in-house committee to the nurses.
5. One-on-one discussions were encouraged.
6. The hospital corrected grossly exaggerated union claims and other inaccuracies by means of a display on their bulletin board in which one column was titled Union Fiction and another was titled Facts. Also, documented handouts stating the hospital's official position on campaign issues and explaining the union's inability to change basic management rights—particularly in the area of scheduling or guaranteeing employees that they couldn't be discharged—were distributed.
7. The hospital encouraged the staff to attend union organizing meetings so that they could be fully informed regarding the union's claims.
8. The nurses were shown sample registered nurse contracts, and the hospital's view of the effects of unionization on the professional practice of nursing was explained.

In these ways, the hospital showed the nurses that their individual freedom, their personal relationships with management, and their professional growth and development would be jeopardized by a union contract. This hospital's campaign, which was aggressive yet sensitive, factual, and balanced, was effective in countering the union's organizing campaign.

HOSPITAL COMMUNICATIONS

It is clear that a health care agency should take an aggressive, positive approach to a union election campaign, rather than simply wait for and react to union handouts and letters. The campaign should be planned with heavy emphasis on timing so that the most potent campaign propaganda appears right before the election. A sample campaign calendar is presented in Exhibit 3-6.

In a union campaign, employers may use any or all of the following:

1. daily bulletin board postings: fact sheets
2. audiovisual materials

Exhibit 3–6 Campaign Calendar

Sunday	Monday	Tuesday	Wednesday	Thursday	Friday	Saturday
	Plan election campaign		Secure LM-2 reports from U.S. Dept. of Labor	Handout: LM-2 report on union organizers' salaries	Movie:[a] Working without unions or We voted no	
	Bulletin board poster: Who would Your Union Steward Be?	Handout: Raise dues notice		Bulletin board poster: 12 Ways a Union Can Get into Your Pocket	Bargaining letter	
	Bulletin board poster: Remember The Last Time You Got Taken?	Handout: Union Dues pie sliced	Bulletin board poster: Weigh the Alternatives	Slide Presentation: Comparison of Present Benefits with Union Contracts	Strike letter, simulated checkoff	
	Bulletin board poster: Be Sure to Vote	Handout: Story of a Strike That Failed		25th hour speech 1:30–2:30 P.M.	Election day Supervisors' election day checklist, handout: How to Vote	Celebrate victory!

[a]The hospital administrator should preview both movies (*Working without unions*, covering blue collar workers, and *We Voted No*, covering office workers) to see which movie fits the employee group being organized.

a. *Working without Unions*, a contemporary film that is the best piece of propaganda released in the last fifteen years for employers fighting a union organizational campaign
    b. *We Voted No*, a videocassette or film for office workers
    c. *Today's Union Organizer*, a study of techniques and ways that the management team may combat organizer tactics, available in film or videocassette
    d. *Union Activity and the Law—The Legal Do's and Don'ts*, a film featuring examples and emphasizing legal rights.[4]
 3. letters to homes on
    a. collective bargaining
    b. strike
    c. staff benefits secured without union dues, fines, or assessments
    d. selected portions of union constitution and bylaws
 4. simulated payroll checkoff insert
 5. one-on-one interviews with employees
 6. handouts (Figure 3–1, Exhibit 3–7)
 7. employee dinners (small group dinners that the hospital pays for)
 8. supervisor's weekly rating of staff based on current information
 9. slide presentation of comparison of other hospital union contracts
 10. twenty-fifth hour speech
 11. election day checklist (Exhibit 3–8)

Fact Sheets

Employers should bring out the facts covering their particular situation in fact sheets. The union constitution could be quoted to show what it takes to secure a strike vote or what is required for trials, fines, and taking the "oath of membership."

In the fact sheets, all employee questions should be answered honestly. A question and answer format may be useful (Exhibit 3–9). The questions and answers should be tailored to the issues that are troubling the staff and should be responsive enough to erase their doubts. Merely posting a number of canned questions and answers is not enough, however. Fact sheets are only starting points for discussions of the real issues in the campaign.

Letters to Homes

Collective Bargaining

One of the letters to the staff should cover the process of collective bargaining. Management should stress that collective bargaining is negotiation and does not

Figure 3–1   Steps Taken by the U.S. Government in Protecting Your Secret
Ballot in an NLRB Election

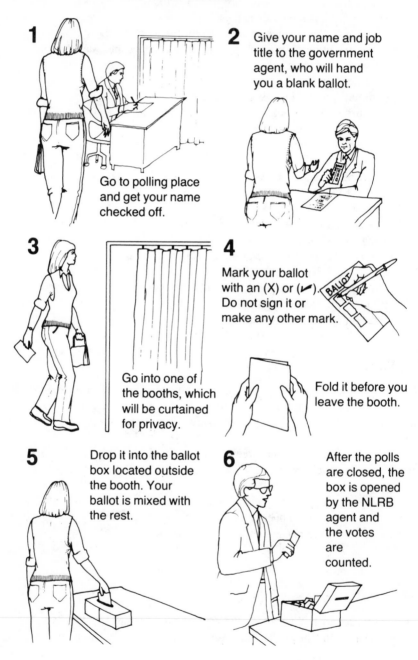

1 Go to polling place and get your name checked off.

2 Give your name and job title to the government agent, who will hand you a blank ballot.

3 Go into one of the booths, which will be curtained for privacy.

4 Mark your ballot with an (X) or (✔). Do not sign it or make any other mark. Fold it before you leave the booth.

5 Drop it into the ballot box located outside the booth. Your ballot is mixed with the rest.

6 After the polls are closed, the box is opened by the NLRB agent and the votes are counted.

Exhibit 3–7 Sample Campaign Literature

IMPORTANT—VOTE ON THE RIGHT SIDE

IF YOU WANT "NO UNION,"

MARK YOUR BALLOT LIKE THIS:_____

BALLOT
NO UNION

ELECTION: Friday, _____
PLACE: _____
TIME: Polls open _____ to _____ P.M.

We are grateful for the loyal support so many of you have indicated to us. We will do everything within our power to justify this support.

Friday, you will at last be able to tell this union how you really feel about it. You will not be left alone *unless* you vote against the union.

The vote will be a secret ballot—no one can ever know how you voted. *Do not sign your ballot.* But remember—*Be sure to vote!* Failure to vote is the same as a "yes" vote for the union, since the union needs only a majority of the votes cast. You can be sure that every would-be union steward will vote! Only if everyone votes will we have the overwhelming majority needed to prove to these outsiders that we want no part of them at XYZ Hospital, now or at any other time! Your vote *is* important, and you should vote to protect yourself.

Vote No   *Vote No*

---

always result in a contract. It should be pointed out that, in *Eastern Maine Medical Center v. NLRB* (lst Cir. 1981) 658 F.2d 1, 92 LC ¶ 12, 981, a court of appeals stated that "the duty to bargain does not compel either party to agree to a proposal or require the making of a concession." The staff should be told that the law says good faith bargaining does not include signing a contract and allows the hospital to reject any demand it feels would jeopardize total patient care. The hospital should not state, however, that "Good faith bargaining does not include signing a contract" without a legal explanation of the bargaining process. It should be added that the

Exhibit 3–8 XYZ Hospital Election Day Checklist

1. Talk to your employees individually, not in groups, from _____ P.M., Thursday, _____, until the election ends on Friday, _____. A group means two or more employees.
2. A schedule of who should vote and when will be circulated.
3. Talk to all employees, especially the fencesitters, because it will be the last person who talks to them who may sway them.
4. All supervisors must stay away from the voting place and make sure that employees who have no business there do not go into the voting area. Be extremely careful that no supervisors or employees talk to employees while they are in line to vote. In other words, there should be no campaigning by anyone (employees or supervisors) while voting is going on.
5. Do not keep a list of employees who have voted. You will be informed of the procedure prior to the election. It probably will be done by department.
6. Make sure employees know that, in order to vote for the hospital and against the union, they must mark an "X" in the NO box on the ballot. Tell your employees not to sign their names or mark up the ballot in any other way.
7. Points to bring out on final contact with employees.
   a. Tell employees who were hired recently of the cost to belong to union—typical cost of dues $180.00 yearly and a typical initiation fee from $25.00 to $150.00.
   b. Emphasize to longer term employees the union's adverse strike record. Violent strikes could happen at XYZ hospital. Also tell them about the stike that failed at _____, in _____, _____.
   c. Union organizer _____, who is attempting to organize our hospital makes $_____ a year (information from LM-2 report secured by your labor attorney) and will be paid even if there is a strike.
   d. The international union will not allow the local employees to run their own show and, in fact, most of the dues money goes to the international union. The _____ union constitution, which provides the oath that employees have to take when they become union members, says all the authority will remain for all intents and purposes with the international union.
   e. Once the union gets in, it is almost impossible to get them out.
   f. Because XYZ Hospital is so small, the union will treat its employees as second class citizens and will not give them the same attention employees at larger hospitals receive.
   g. During a strike, employees not only lose wages, but their hospitalization insurance is terminated and they are not eligible for unemployment compensation!!!
   h. If employees go on strike, the hospital has a legal right to keep operating and intends to exercise this right. To do this, the hospital can hire permanent replacements for each and every employee. When this happens, employees lose their jobs and are put on "a preferential hiring list."
   i. The union is a big business and is not really interested in the problems of XYZ Hospital employees but is only interested in the money that they get in dues.
8. On election day thank the employees for their support. Let them know that you feel it will be an overwhelming victory for the hospital. Tell them you are counting on them and remind them to Vote No!!!

Exhibit 3–9 Fact Sheet

Q: Won't the union obtain higher wages or the "standard union rate" if we vote it in?

A: The union can promise anything, but it cannot guarantee anything. There are no such things as standard union rates. The hospital is paying as much as other hospitals in this area are paying and, union or no union, will continue to do so. Wages are negotiable, and the hospital does not have to agree to any demand it feels is unreasonable.

Q: Won't the hospital be forced to sign a union contract if the union gets in?

A: The hospital's only duty under the law is to bargain in good faith. The law does not require the hospital to sign a contract or agree to any demand it feels is unreasonable. The only weapon a union has against the hospital is a strike. Many times a union never secures a contract.

Q: Won't the union secure a formal grievance and arbitration procedure if voted in?

A: The union cannot even guarantee this. Actually, there are an increasing number of cases in which employees are suing their own union because the union refused to handle their grievances. Furthermore, the union steward may decide to settle your grievance on terms that you do not like or to trade your grievance to resolve another matter. They may trade what is important to employees in order to gain union security, such as a union shop or an automatic dues checkoff. Also, a grievance takes an average of six months to one year to go through arbitration. Here you receive an answer in hours or, at the most, in two or three days.

Q: Won't the union provide job security?

A: Unions cannot ensure a favorable business climate, which is the only thing that provides job security. All union contracts with which we are familiar provide for discharges, layoffs, and shutdowns.

Q: Won't the union give me the power to tell management what to do and to fire unpopular supervisors?

A: No. The union cannot force the hospital to do anything that it feels is not in its best interest. Every union contract we have heard of has a management rights clause that gives management the right to run the hospital, including the right to hire and fire. If you would like to see samples of such union contract clauses, we would be happy to show them to you.

Q: How much are the union's dues?

A: Union dues can run to hundreds of dollars a year. Furthermore, the union can raise dues without consulting its members. It can assess you to pay for a strike at another hospital. It can fine you for not attending union meetings, for refusing to join a strike, for informing management that a fellow union member violated a house rule, and for making derogatory remarks about the union. Most of the money from dues and fines goes to the international union for the salaries and expense accounts of union officials. A typical union constitution clause provides for the "prompt" payment of assessments and fines in order to remain in good standing, as follows: "A member shall . . . continue to pay all dues, assessments, and fines or other obligations promptly when due in order to be and remain in good standing."

Exhibit 3–9 continued

Q: If there is a strike, won't I get strike benefits from the union's strike fund?

A: Many unions have very little in a strike fund as hardly any of the members' dues are placed in such a fund. Also, typical strike benefits are twenty-five to thirty dollars a week and are paid only to those who walk the picket line.

Q: If there is a strike, doesn't the hospital have to give me my old job back after the strike is over?

A: The law states that the hospital has the legal right to continue its services, even if there is a strike. When you strike for a contract, the hospital can hire a permanent replacement for you, and you cannot have your job back until your replacement leaves, which could be a very long time.

Q: Can't the union guarantee all my present benefits?

A: The union cannot guarantee *any* benefit. In fact, it could trade some of your present benefits to obtain clauses for union security (not employee security), a union shop, and a checkoff clause. Your present benefits are secured only if the hospital is strong and healthy and only if financial conditions justify them.

Q: What do I have to lose by joining the union?

A: We feel that we now have a forum for a healthy interchange of ideas between staff and management. Bringing in an outside third party interferes with your ability to participate as an individual in making decisions about the working conditions as they affect you. As your representative, the union would exercise that function, thereby eliminating the type of participatory management we now enjoy.

Q: Why is the hospital campaigning so strongly against the union?

A: A union will not help us provide better patient care, and in our opinion, it will destroy the professional and harmonious atmosphere we all enjoy. We feel the union would create a "war zone" where employees dread coming to work. The union may tell you there will never be a strike; however, a strike is the union's only weapon, and everyone must assume it will be used. Patients will not understand your walking out on them in the event of a strike. We feel that a union would prevent the staff and management from providing a total health care approach for patient care.

hospital will negotiate in good faith and that the letter's author is merely expressing a personal opinion of bargaining.

The letter should also bring out that, although individuals are led to believe that bargaining starts at the *present* level of employee wages and fringe benefits, this is not true. Everything is negotiable, including present wages and fringe benefits. The NLRB said in *Midwestern Instruments, Inc.*, 133 NLRB 1132 (1961), that "there is, of course, no obligation on the part of an employer to contract to continue all existing benefits, nor is it an unfair labor practice to offer reduced benefits." The hospital should not make the statement that bargaining starts from "zero" or from "scratch," although it may state that bargaining starts from a minimum proposal."

It should also be made clear in the letter that management does not have to give up any of its basic management rights, such as those in the area of scheduling, if it feels that this is not in the best interests of the health care agency and its patients. The staff should be told that the union knows this, but will not tell them. For an example of a sample letter explaining collective bargaining, see Exhibit 3-10.

Strikes

In its communications on strikes, the hospital must not suggest that a strike is inevitable (see *Dominican Santa Cruz Hospital,* 242 NLRB No. 153 [1979]). The staff can be told, however, that employees who strike for wages receive neither their salaries nor unemployment compensation (in most states) and that the hospital is legally entitled to stop making payments on their medical, hospital, and life insurance premiums.

The union may counter by saying that a strike has not even been mentioned. That will probably be true. The union wants to hide the fact that its only weapon when negotiations fail is to call a strike. The staff should not accept unionism if they do not approve of strikes.

In the aftermath of an actual strike, the following illuminating post-strike reaction was given by striking nurses. At the beginning of the strike, the nurses were boisterous and handed out handbills claiming that patients were being subjected to unsafe conditions such as medication errors because of the lack of qualified personnel. Blocked entrances were creating hazards until the hospital obtained an injunction limiting the number of pickets and continued admitting patients. After the strike was over, the nurses were severely criticized by the patients and the patients' families for deserting them in their hour of need. The nurses stated that the strike was a highly emotional experience and that they felt guilty in facing their patients and the patients' families because of their disapproval of the nurses' deserting them.

An example of a letter conveying the consequences of a strike is shown in Exhibit 3-11.

Twenty-Fifth Hour Speech

Management should begin the twenty-fifth hour speech by summarizing the hospital's accomplishments to date without a union. The speaker should:

- point out the many contributions the hospital has made in the professional development of the staff, in continuing education, and in the area of wages and fringe benefits
- emphasize the ways that management and staff have shared decision making to make patient care excellent

Exhibit 3–10 Collective Bargaining Letter

Dear Staff:

You and the hospital are faced with a union organizing attempt, and we are writing to you today to ask your understanding, support, and cooperation. In fairness to you, we want you to know how strongly we feel that we do not need a union here and that this union would jeopardize your professional development, as well as the participatory management and collaborative decision making that the staff and the hospital management now enjoy.

The union makes it sound so easy: demand and you will receive. This is absolutely wrong! It is easy to make promises, but the union cannot deliver. The hospital can, but we are going to promise you only that we will remain competitive in wages and fringe benefits.

If the union wins, all it can do is to sit at the bargaining table. There is a common misconception that, if the union wins the election, a contract is automatically signed and wages and fringe benefits are automatically improved. However, this is not the case. Negotiations often go on for many months. In fact, it could be months or years before negotiations even begin or before any contract is reached.

The truth is that bargaining starts from a minimum proposal. The union salesman usually wants a union shop and a dues checkoff and could very well trade some of your present benefits, such as insurance, sick days, or holidays, for these clauses. The professional union salesman would like you to believe you have nothing to lose and everything to gain. However, you have your current individual rights to bargain for wages, scheduling, choice of work areas, decisions on continuing education, and orientation of staff that the union may bargain away. These day-to-day rights that you have to share in the decision-making process as it affects your job may be gone forever.

Also, when you embrace the concept of unionism, you embrace the union's only weapon to get the hospital to agree to anything—a strike. In our bargaining, if the union does not like our answers to their demands, they can take you out on strike. In this event, the hospital legally can continue to operate and maintain its census at the level prior to the strike. In order to accomplish this, it may permanently replace economic strikers, who would then be placed on a preferential hiring list and who may or may not have a job after the strike is over. More importantly, ask yourselves how could you face your patients if you strike and deprive them of necessary patient care.

So we ask you again for your continued support and understanding. All we ask is a chance to work together. For everyone's benefit—yours, your family's, the hospital's, and our patients'— we strongly urge you not to be influenced by these outsiders who are interested only in your monthly union dues, not in better care for our patients.

Now, when the health care industry is in such a difficult economic time and we are all lucky to have jobs, we need to pull together as a team, without strikes, dues, and initiation fees, for our mutual success.

The only answer is to vote NO on ___(date)___ .

Sincerely,

Exhibit 3–11 Strike Letter

Dear Staff:

    Is a vote for a union the same as a vote for a strike? This is a most serious question, and we are not sure of the answer. We feel that it is our duty to tell you about this union's strike record. It is our considered opinion that if this union gets in, it would be possible for a very small group of union militants to take you out on strike!

    A few of our more militant employees have indicated that they want the union so that it could "force" us to do things. Let me assure you that we will not be forced to do anything that is not in the best interest of this hospital, its patients, and the entire staff. Stop and think what these militant employees, who would be on the union committee to deal with management, might do in an attempt to force us to agree to something we believed was unreasonable. The union's constitution and bylaws provide that, if at least two-thirds of those voting at a meeting called for that purpose vote to strike, the president shall direct and call a strike. Therefore, if only nine employees attend such a meeting, only six employees who want a strike could take you out on strike.

    If there is a strike, there are some very important facts you should know:

1. If a strike occurs, you stop earning wages immediately.
2. The hospital can legally stop making medical, hospital, and life insurance premium payments.
3. You would not be eligible for unemployment insurance, as our state does not pay unemployment compensation for strikers.
4. The union will pay, maybe, $25.00 to $30.00 a week in strike benefits if you walk the picket line. Could you exist on $25.00 a week?
5. You can lose your job when you go out on strike. The hospital has the right to continue operations and hire permanent replacements.

    Although a strike is not inevitable, we believe that you will be deciding on election day whether you will be placed in a situation that could lead to strikes, picket lines, loss of patient respect for striking staff members, and even violence.

    We would bargain in good faith to reach an agreement, but we feel no employee should be forced to join a union. The union's insistence on a union shop and unreasonable demands could lead to a strike.

    Would the union call a strike at this hospital? We do not know! The union says that you decide whether to strike, but the union controls every strike vote. We urge all of you to examine this union's strike record; the attached sheets list just some of their strikes since 1978.

    We do not believe that you want to gamble with your professional development or your career or, most importantly, with the health and welfare of our patients and bring into the hospital a union that could lead to strikes, picket lines, and violence.

    The future is really up to you. Protect yourself and your fellow staff members by voting no in the election on ____(date)____ .

    We started this letter by asking if a vote for the union is the same as a vote for a strike. Isn't the best answer to vote no on election day!

Sincerely,

(Health Care Institution)

_____

(Administrator)

- emphasize the importance of a multidisciplinary team approach and how an outside party would add confusion to efforts in this area
- discuss the hospital's effort to improve scheduling and point out the complexity of scheduling and how a union cannot make scheduling problems disappear
- explain the hospital's view of the effects of unionization on professional practice, emphasizing the drawbacks
- show how the union would not facilitate the delivery of better patient care, but in fact, would seriously hinder it
- explain the individual rights and power lost by blindly assigning power to a union as the exclusive representative
- explain the bargaining process, the fact that the union is not liable for keeping promises that it makes in the campaign, and that the staff could lose present wages and benefits as a result of collective bargaining
- explain what the employees are agreeing to when they *swear* to uphold the union's constitution and bylaws
- raise questions such as
  1. Can the union call a strike without a vote by secret ballot?
  2. What can the union fine its members for?
  3. How much can the union charge for initiation fees and dues?
  4. Can the union raise dues without approval of the membership?
  5. What is the limit on the amount of dues that a union can charge?
  6. In the event of a strike, what provisions does the union make for paying members' bills and continuing their insurance?
- present facts on the union in other hospitals
- make it clear that the union can fine them for crossing a picket line, even though their intent is to provide care for critically ill patients
- emphasize that the union cannot guarantee special shifts or time off on weekends or holidays
- explain that others will have to do the work of the area representative if that representative is called away for union business, giving an illustration of the difficulty this could cause at peak hours of the shift
- give an example of the red tape required when an employee registers a complaint with the union so that the union becomes the third party in employee communication with management
- tell employees that the hospital cannot be forced to sign a contract or to agree to any unreasonable union demands and that the only weapon the union has is a strike
- point out that unions cost hospitals a great deal of money that could be spent on employees and patient services (most experts agree that a union increases

hospital costs 20 to 25 percent with no corresponding increase in productivity)

- explain that the forum for healthy interchange of ideas between management and employees is severely undercut by a union, which must pit management against employees to create a war zone of mistrust to justify its existence
- tell employees to think about the ethical implications of leaving sick patients to go out on strike, giving factual examples of what patients think and feel when hospital employees, especially nurses, walk out
- emphasize the fact that the union uses a strike as a weapon and that acceptance of the union means employees have to accept the possibility of strike

If there are so many disadvantages to unionization, then *why* do employees turn to a union? From an analysis of many unionization campaigns, the following list of the more important reasons that employees look to unionization and sign authorization cards was compiled:

1. Unfair and harsh treatment by immediate supervisors. Employees believe they can get even with management for real or imaginary wrongs and failure to listen to them.
2. Little, if any, personal recognition.
3. Lack of fair, firm, and consistent discipline.
4. Job insecurity.
5. Failure of management to exercise confident leadership.
6. Unsatisfactory complaint procedure.
7. Failure of management to help employees identify with the hospital. Employees believe they will have the opportunity to "participate" in the satisfaction of their personal needs through union membership.
8. Favoritism.
9. Lack of or inadequate employee benefits.
10. Substandard wages.
11. Failure of management to put hospital personnel policies and employee benefits in writing.
12. Lack of recognition for length of service on the job.
13. Verbal abuse of employees.
14. Failure of management to "sell" the employees on the benefits and advantages of working for the hospital.
15. Feelings of frustration and boredom.

Important Caveat: Card-Based Bargaining Orders

Hospitals should be aware that a union can become the bargaining representative of their employees even when it loses an NLRB secret ballot election. At the time of *Aiello Dairy Farms,* 35 LRRM 1235 (1954), the Board would not entertain post-election refusal-to-bargain charges by a defeated union on the ground that the union, when it determined the employer had engaged in unfair labor practices, had to choose between proving its majority in the election and filing a refusal-to-bargain charge. In *Bernel Foam Products Co.,* 56 LRRM 1309 (1964), however, the NLRB decided that henceforth it would entertain refusal-to-bargain charges based on the employer's failure to recognize the union prior to the election, even if the union lost the election, assuming it could prove its majority status at the time it demanded recognition.

This procedure was further clarified in 1969 when the U.S. Supreme Court heard several cases in which the NLRB had issued bargaining orders on the ground that the employer's refusal to recognize the union had been motivated not by a "good faith doubt" of the union's majority status but by a desire to gain time to dissipate that status. The Court, in the landmark case of *NLRB v. Gissel Packing Co.,* 395 U.S. 585 (1969), held that an employer's good faith doubt was irrelevant and that the key to a bargaining order was the commission of serious (flagrant) unfair labor practices that interfere with the election process and preclude a fair election. Simply stated, the Court held in *Gissel* that a bargaining obligation may be created even without an election victory if the union represents a majority of the involved employees, which is usually the case when the union proceeds to an election. The Court also approved the Board's acceptance of union authorization cards to prove majority support, as the cards may be the only reliable proof of such support when the employer has impeded the election process by committing serious unfair labor practices.

The NLRB determines if the unfair labor practices preclude a fair election. In *General Stencils, Inc.,* 195 NLRB No. 173 (1972) 79 LRRM 1608, Chairman Edward B. Miller in a dissenting opinion gave a well-reasoned model of the unfair labor practices that, in his opinion, preclude a fair election. Of course, granting a wage increase just before the election to satisfy the employees' demands rather than one conforming to a past practice would be considered a serious unfair labor practice. Discharging the main union adherents in a small bargaining unit should also qualify as an unfair practice that would preclude a fair election and result in a bargaining order based on union authorization cards. Threatening to close the hospital rather than bargain with a union is also in this category.

Even though the union has not sent the employer a formal demand letter, the Board has held that the election petition itself constitutes a demand for recognition. In some very rare cases in which the employer totally rejects the NLRA and flagrantly violates it, the Board has held not only that the union does not need to have sent a demand for recognition, but also that the union does not even have to be a majority-selected union! In *Conair Corp.,* 261 NLRB No. 178 (1982), the Board ordered an employer in such circumstances (flagrant unfair labor practices) to bargain with a minority representative. However, the Court of Appeals of the

District of Columbia refused to enforce this nonmajority bargaining order holding that the NLRB lacks authority under the Taft-Hartley Act "to issue a bargaining order absent a concrete manifestation of majority support for the union." See *Conair Corporation v. NLRB* (D.C. Cir. 1983) No. 223 DLR November 17, 1983, A-10, text D-1.

The employer must insist on an election and must not agree to some other form of ascertaining the union's majority status, such as a union authorization card check by some alleged neutral third party. Employers who agree to this or who ask for and receive the cards for their own verification cannot reject the finding of majority representation if that is what the cards show. Many times, however, union authorization cards are misrepresented as to their purpose, signed to get rid of a union official, or signed at a time when peer pressure interfered with the employee's true feelings; union authorization cards are not reliable indicators of majority support. Similarly, the results of an oral poll cannot be rejected. Thus, the right to a secret ballot election is lost.

ELECTION OUTCOME

During the election campaign, consistent quiet among the employees who will vote is usually a bad sign. A healthy debate in which management has honestly and openly taken the offensive and has grass roots support from respected staff members is a very good sign. Employee questions toward the end of the campaign about what will happen to staff members who supported the union if the union loses suggest that the union will lose the election. If the positive campaign strategies previously mapped out are followed, with management being aggressive but fair, a successful campaign will be achieved and the hospital will maintain its union-free status.

NOTES

1. Disclosure Bureau, Labor Management Services Administration U.S. Department of Labor, 200 Constitution Avenue, N.W., Washington, DC 20216.

2. Office of Labor-Management and Welfare-Pension Reports, Publications Department, 8701 Georgia Avenue, Silver Spring, MD 20910.

3. Bureau of National Affairs, Inc., Special Projects Division, 1231 Twenty-fifth Street, N.W., Washington, DC 20037.

4. All these films can be obtained by calling 1-800-554-1389 or writing Thompson-Mitchell and Associates, 3384 Peachtree Road, N.E., Atlanta, GA 30326.

Chapter 4

Collective Bargaining Negotiations

The process of contract negotiations has been compared to a poker game, but managers would be foolhardy to regard it as such. These negotiation sessions are serious meetings in which the success of a hospital as a business and the future of its employees are determined. Moreover, these meetings determine management rights in the daily operation of health care services. For these reasons, the members of the management negotiating team must be carefully selected on the basis of their collective bargaining experience and their knowledge of the particular hospital.[1,2]

This team must gather all pertinent data and articulate the positions of the union and of the hospital on points of compromise or firm stands on issues. Finally, they must outline their strategy based on knowledge of the union, the hospital, the issues, the demands, and the strengths and weaknesses of the hospital position. An analysis of campaign issues in the organizational effort and contract provisions at hospitals where the union is involved is critical to the formulation of management's strategy. Other major items to study include

- problems and issues arising during the administration of the existing contract
- costs of implementing contract provisions
- grievance and arbitration issues, decisions, and precedents
- issues identified by department heads in special prenegotiation meetings
- position of the board of directors on potential issues
- guidelines for the power and functional operation of the negotiating team and the chief spokespersons
- competition in wages and fringe benefits in the area[3]

The management team should attempt to obtain a copy of the union demands prior to bargaining and should review these demands with the hospital's labor attorney to ensure that they comply with the legal and accrediting demands imposed on the hospital. They must also determine whether the union has complied with legal procedures to make negotiations possible. The management team needs to review its own proposals to be certain that they contain no violations of new laws or standards of practice that could undermine the hospital's reputation, legal status, or ability to provide quality care to patients.[4]

Management should prepare a memo to present to the union during the first meeting. For example,

> In working toward a contractual agreement, we reserve the right during negotiations to substitute proposals for those initially presented and to add or to delete proposals as negotiations proceed.
>
> It is our position that no final agreement is binding on particular sections of the contract until a total agreement on all portions of the contract is reached and ratified. We understand that tentative agreement on specific items will probably occur as proposals are considered. These tentative agreements, however, will be final only after the hospital's board of directors has approved them.
>
> We request written notification on the extent of authority of the union bargainers. Please state membership ratification requirements, if any. The hospital will furnish the same information to the union.

Management negotiators should then carefully consider all points on a checklist similar to that shown in Exhibit 4–1.

THE HOSPITAL TEAM

The directors of personnel, nursing, finance, and public relations, as well as the associate hospital director and appropriate representatives from the affected bargaining unit, should be included on the hospital team. The chief spokesperson should be an experienced labor law attorney or professional labor negotiator who has been involved in a number of labor negotiation sessions for hospitals. The chief executive officer should not be at the table because the absence of this officer (1) allows the management team to take time to consider decisions rationally and deliberately while discussing them with the chief executive officer (2) prevents the union from using the chief executive officer's reactions as a barometer, and (3) provides a reasonable excuse for the team to caucus with appropriate others, such as the board of directors or various department heads, to gather necessary factual data.

Exhibit 4–1 Checklist for Collective Bargaining Negotiations

The Hospital Committee

1. Prepare a list of the members of the negotiating committee showing

   - name
   - title
   - business address and telephone number
   - home address and telephone number
   - temporary address and telephone number (if staying in a hotel, for example, during negotiations).

2. Make sure that each member has a telephone number where urgent messages can be left between meetings.
3. Ascertain whether the offices and telephones for the committee are "secure" for sensitive information.
4. Prepare similar lists for all backup personnel who may have to be contacted for information during negotiations.
5. Appoint a spokesperson to do the actual talking at the table.
6. Appoint a committee member to take detailed notes during negotiations.
7. Appoint one member to be responsible for ensuring that all notes and documents are removed from the bargaining room during caucuses.
8. Instruct the secretaries and assistants of all committee members not to disturb them for nonemergency matters during negotiations.
9. Consider whether the company official with the actual authority to agree to a proposal should be a member of the committee.
10. Establish the exact limits of the committee's authority to accept and reject union proposals.

The Union Committee

1. Determine the names of the union committee members, and prepare a list of their addresses and telephone numbers.
3. Ascertain, if possible, what union factions will be represented at the table and who will be influential with these factions during bargaining.
3. Analyze any special problems or opportunities presented by the union committee members, such as

   - animosity toward the company or the company committee members
   - special friendships or obligations toward company committee members
   - possibility of confidential or off-the-record negotiations or discussions with the union committee members.

Preparation for Negotiations

1. Meet with supervisors and executives to evaluate experience under the expiring contract; review policies, procedures, and current practices; and gather suggestions for contract changes.
2. Analyze grievances and subjects of discontent.
3. Try to ascertain what employees really want in upcoming negotiations.

Exhibit 4-1 continued

4. Evaluate past and anticipated future problems arising from existing contract language in light of production and administrative plans, prior arbitration awards, union positions taken in past controversies, and any available information concerning union plans and goals.

5. Analyze the expiring contract terms to determine which terms

   - are still acceptable to the hospital
   - the hospital wants to change
   - the union may want to change.

6. Establish the hospital's position with regard to

   - the length of the new contract
   - union shops
   - dues checkoff
   - cost of living clause.

7. Determine whether it is possible simply to renew the same contract, without change, and negotiate only on the wages.

8. Analyze the union's current power politics to determine who actually controls the union and who is most influential among the bargaining unit members.

9. Brief all committee members on the union's proposals and the hospital's proposals.

10. Outline problem areas and sensitive issues.

11. Brief committee members on the hospital's bargaining objectives.

12. Ensure that committee members understand they should not make unguarded statements at the table or during recesses and that the spokesperson should do all the talking.

13. Provide each committee member with a notebook containing hospital and union proposals, as well as grievances and arbitration decisions, cross-referenced to contract clauses and bargaining data.

14. Collect copies of contracts with the union, particularly those negotiated by the same international representative, after the expiring contract was signed.

15. Collect copies of other union contracts or policies of comparable hospitals in the area.

16. Obtain national and local cost-of-living indexes for last year and present year.[5]

17. Prepare list in three columns of

Present Contract Clause	Desired Company Changes	Reason for Changes

18. In four columns prepare list of

Present Contract Clause	Union Demand for Change	Company Position (Strike Issue)	Estimate of Cost If Changes Granted

19. Write a description of every job classification and its present wage rate, classifying costs as direct, indirect, and total costs.

20. Prepare a survey comparable wage rates and fringe benefits of competitors in industry and area, including only those jobs and wage rates that closely match those of the hospital.

Exhibit 4–1 continued

21. Calculate the average gross (overtime), including hourly and weekly earnings of those in the bargaining unit.
22. Calculate the average amount of overtime per week.
23. List the cost of present fringe benefits, including indirect costs such as Social Security, Workmen's Compensation, unemployment insurance, payroll, taxes, wages paid for time spent on union activity.

	Average Hourly Cost		
Fringe Benefits	Direct	Indirect	Total
Paid holidays			
Paid vacations			
Paid insurance			
Paid sick leave			
Premium pay			
Shift difference			
Jury duty			
Funeral leave			

24. List the number of employees with continuous service of one year, two years, three years, five years, ten years, fifteen years, and twenty-five years.
25. Calculate the average age of those in bargaining unit, where applicable.
26. Estimate the cost of granting each union demand.
27. Estimate the cost of company proposals.
28. Estimate approximately the maximum limit that the hospital can grant and remain competitive.
29. List pertinent recent wage settlements with the union in the community and industry.
30. Consider the language of clauses in other contracts that the union has in the area that are favorable to the hospital.
31. Obtain the current seniority list.
32. Estimate hourly cost of union demands.

	Cents per Hour		
Union Demand	Avg. Increment	Indirect	Total

33. List arguments against union demands.
34. List wages, benefits, and Contract conditions of competitors and employers hiring similarly skilled employees.
35. Average hourly wage of similarly skilled employees.
36. Calculate the average number of hours worked per year (last three years) by all employees in the bargaining unit.
37. Calculate the average number of hours worked per year by job classification (for last three years).
38. Calculate the labor in percentage terms to total revenue (productivity), i.e., total cost of labor divided by total revenue.
39. Calculate the capital investment in dollar figures per employee.

Meeting Arrangements

1. Select a suitable meeting place, such as a hotel or other neutral location.
2. Arrange for a table and chairs for all participants.

Exhibit 4–1 continued

3. Make sure the room is large enough to spread out and still keep notes confidential.
4. Arrange for a telephone in the room.
5. Arrange for caucus rooms, with telephones for both hospital and union negotiators.
6. Arrange with the union to split the cost of rooms and room service.
7. Consider whether coffee and snacks should be provided.
8. Check whether the caucus rooms are vulnerable to eavesdropping.
9. Ensure adequate lighting and ventilation in all rooms.
10. Check for adequate eating and restroom facilities nearby.
11. Try to arrange a break area, with refreshment machines and upholstered chairs for stretch breaks.
12. Decide with the union

   • whether meetings will be during or after work
   • whether the hospital will pay the union committee members for any time spent in negotiations
   • length of sessions
   • frequency of sessions
   • caucus calls and arrangements
   • breaks
   • exchange of proposals.

13. Determine who, e.g., the membership for the union and the board of directors for the hospital, must approve the agreement reached at the table.
14. Make clear that bargaining is for an entire agreement, and the clauses can be renegotiated if new proposals are made.

The personnel and finance directors are at the table because of their obvious expertise in the areas to be discussed. The director of nursing usually represents a majority of employees in the hospital and is a good representative to have at the table. The director of public relations is a part of the proceedings to handle communications sent to employees and news releases to the media. The associate administrator represents a high authority of the hospital, although not the ultimate one.

Members of the management team must be well aware of the process and legal aspects of collective bargaining and must be completely prepared to endure the challenges, frustrations, disappointments, and tactics inherent in negotiating a settlement. The team must be well disciplined. Only the chief negotiator presents and argues points in the proposal. Other team members do not usually speak unless they have prior permission of the chief negotiator. The team must present an air of solidarity so that differences among team members do not become obvious to the union negotiating team.

THE BARGAINING OBLIGATION

Before any contract negotiations, the labor law attorney and the hospital administrator determine whether they are lawfully obligated to bargain with the employee representative. In first contracts, bargaining representatives of the majority of employees can be determined in only three ways:

1. The union may have won an election conducted by the National Labor Relations Board (NLRB).
2. The union may have "come in on the cards." When flagrant unfair labor practices negate the holding of a free and uncoerced election, the Board may nullify the election. This procedure is known as Gisselling the election. The Board may order that the union be recognized as the majority representative of the employees if they show that a majority of the employees in the appropriate bargaining unit signed union authorization cards when the union demanded recognition.
3. The employer may voluntarily recognize the union. This can occur when the union representative shows the administrator the union authorization cards, and the administrator agrees to be bound by this method. To avoid this problem, administrators are told to avoid looking at these cards from the union and to avoid making any such agreements until they are legally required to do so.

Notice Periods

Before an existing contract is re-negotiated, administrators must determine that the contract is legally open to such negotiations and that the party wishing to modify, bargain, or amend the contract has given the stipulated notice. Some contracts are automatically renewed from year to year when timely notice is not given. If the contract expires on its own terms, the hospital is required to negotiate a new contract only if the union retains its majority status as bargaining agent of the employees.

Good Faith Bargaining

An employer must bargain with the union for one full year after the time of its certification as the majority representative of the employees. While there are a few unusual circumstances that alter this obligation, changes in the loyalties or sentiments of employees are not a reason to cease bargaining during the certification year. Bargaining obligations beyond the year of certification depend on the union's ability to maintain its status as the majority representative of the employees. If a majority of employees in the appropriate bargaining unit sign a petition stating they do not want the union to represent them, the employer can withdraw recognition if no contract is in effect. This is assuming that the employer did not solicit, urge, or sponsor such a petition.

The National Labor Relations Act (NLRA) is very specific on the obligations of both parties to bargain. While good faith bargaining is required of both, the NLRA does not demand that such negotiations end in a written contract. In first contracts, the parties are bound to (1) meet at reasonable times to negotiate wages, hours, and other terms and conditions of employment in good faith, namely with an intent to reach an agreement; and (2) place into writing and execute a contract stipulating agreements that have been reached.

The NLRB looks at total conduct in the context of the bargaining relationship to justify bad faith bargaining charges. While no set number of meetings is required, the Board carefully considers the number of meetings, the substantive nature of the meetings, the initiative of the employer in scheduling meetings, and the delays or cancellations of meetings. In making arrangements or sending documents and minutes, a hospital should ensure that everything is written and sent to the union by certified mail. Such documentation is essential in defending the management team against a potential charge of refusal to bargain.

The Board tends to find that the employer must be available for negotiations once or twice a week, particularly when negotiating for a first contract. When a hospital's management team is passive and unavailable, the certification year may be extended to make up for the period in which the hospital bargained in bad faith. Furthermore, the union may strike over the employer's unilateral actions on mandatory subjects of bargaining or the infrequency of the meetings. This strike would be an unfair labor practice strike, wherein strikers could *not* be permanently replaced. These strikers would have to be reinstated and their replacements discharged.

Hard Bargaining

A "take it or leave it" attitude is inappropriate at the bargaining table, as determined in the famous case of *General Electric Co.*, 150 NLRB 192 (1964). Employers must not seem inflexible when they present demands that the NLRB defines as inherently objectionable to the union. An unwillingness to compromise violates the spirit and intent of good faith bargaining. Each party must exhibit an *intent* to reach agreement by the totality of its conduct.

Even though Section 8(d) of the NLRA says that the employer is not required to make any concessions, the Board penalizes those who do not make concessions during the bargaining process. The leading case on whether the Board can order an employer to make a concession is *H.K. Porter Co. v. NLRB*, 397 U.S. 99, 90 S. Ct. 821 (1970). In this case, the Supreme Court held that the Board could not order the employer to agree to the union's demand for a dues checkoff clause. This reasoning would apply to other clauses, such as union shop, management rights, seniority, promotions, and shift scheduling. If in all these areas no concessions are made, however, the Board may find that the employer is attempting to operate as if no union existed and may rule that this is unlawful bad faith bargaining, not legal hard bargaining.

Given this quandry, the employer must decide which major areas are of such grave concern that no concessions can be made and which major areas, such as shift scheduling procedure, allow flexibility. For example, one hospital made a scheduling arrangement that included a provision to "discuss" new ideas with the union. Thus, the hospital agreed to "discuss" how to utilize flexitime scheduling to meet area staffing shortages or to staff in circumstances unforeseen during contract negotiations. The hospital did, in fact, make a concession in a very important area.

There is a fine line between hard bargaining and bad faith bargaining. Various contractual demands may be made by the employer in showing intent to reach an agreement without compromising the employer's best interests. Such skillful and artful negotiating requires knowledge about the specific hospital, health care labor relations, and a wealth of experience at the bargaining table.[6,7]

Renewal of Contracts

Negotiations are the same for contract renewals as for first contracts, except that the parties are expected to utilize the existing contract as a basis for negotiation unless they have legitimate business reasons to modify or delete particular clauses.

During the existence of a contract, administrators should compile a grievance list on each clause of the contract. This indexed list should include problems of interpretation, implementation, and points arising from grievances and arbitrations.[8,9]

SUBJECTS OF BARGAINING

Wages, hours, and other terms and conditions of employment are mandatory subjects of bargaining. Typical items included in this category are

- recognition of the union
- management rights
- no strike, no lockout clause
- union security
- wages
- dues checkoff

- seniority
- scheduling
- promotions, job bidding
- leaves of absence
- holidays
- vacations
- sick leave
- personal leave
- union representation, i.e., number of stewards
- grievance and arbitration procedure
- health and welfare insurance
- change in employee status
- change in job classifications
- changes in hours
- merit increases
- nondiscrimination
- employee obligations and duties clause
- shift differential
- separability and savings, i.e., if one clause is held illegal, the rest of the contract remains valid and
- length and termination of the contract

The union liability clause must also be discussed. The trend in collective bargaining in the 1980s is to make the union liable in those areas in which it wants to have voice. For example, if the union wants to inspect a hospital for health and safety hazards, they should be held jointly responsible and jointly liable for any employee injury, illness, or death. This is premised on the concept that joint action requires joint liability in any clause.

Permissible subjects of bargaining might include benefits for retirees, a strike liability bond for breaches of the no strike clause, and the mechanics of the ratification of the contract vote (i.e., secret ballot). These items rarely come up for discussion, however. Unlike a mandatory subject, permissible topics may not be advanced to the point of impasse or strike.

Pet Clauses of the Union

Russian Veto. Clauses that require management to obtain the union's agreement before taking an action are called Russian veto clauses. For example, an employee will lose seniority for absenteeism upon agreement of both the hospital and the union.

Supervisor Working Clause. A union often wants a clause that prohibits anyone except those in the bargaining unit from performing bargaining unit work. This clause keeps a physician from giving an aspirin or a routine medication to a patient. Clearly, this clause can cause numerous problems.

Supervisors in the Union. The hospital does not have to agree that supervisors must become union members. However, if supervisors are excluded from the unit and the supervisor working clause, which prohibits those excluded from the bargaining unit from doing bargaining unit work, has been agreed upon, supervisors will not be able to function as required in the life and death, unpredictable environment of the hospital, Therefore, management needs a sentence stating that all supervisors and other managers who are not part of the certified bargaining unit can do any and all work that they did in the past. A union may not strike to force an employer to agree that supervisors become union members, since this is a permissible subject of bargaining.

Maintenance of Standards. The hospital may want a clause such as

> The hospital agrees to maintain all standards of employment, including wages, hours, and working conditions or terms of employment, at not less than the highest standards in effect when this agreement is signed. The conditions of employment shall be improved wherever specific provisions are made in other parts of this agreement.[10]

Signing this clause is paramount to buying a "pig in a poke." The hospital is agreeing to standards, some of which it may not even be aware. Standards that are important to employees must be negotiated individually so that everyone knows what they are. Also, such a clause freezing the status quo is undesirable, because it could hinder improvements in the conditions affecting the hospital, its employees, and its patients.

Subcontracting. The hospital's agreement to give up its fundamental right to subcontract work, even though it could be performed by hospital employees, could interfere with the basic conduct of business operations. For example, this clause could become a problem when the hospital is remodeling an area, contracting out emergency services or vehicle agreements, sending away laboratory studies, or using another facility to perform rehabilitation services. Furthermore, someone must determine when hospital employees are actually available to do the work. This clause could require the hospital to maintain a service that is no longer needed but is expensive and inefficient. For the success of the business, the hospital must determine who is going to produce what product or service.

In opposition to the union's clause, the hospital should frame a management rights clause so that the union waives its right to bargain on subcontracting. The following is recommended:

> The management of the hospital, the control of the premises, and the direction of the work force are vested exclusively with the hospital. The right to manage includes, but shall not be limited to, the right to hire, transfer, promote, lay off, and suspend or discharge employees for just cause; to specify or alter the shifts and the number of hours to be worked by employees; to change shifts or establish additional or new shifts, temporary or permanent, in any department at any time and transfer any employee from one schedule of hours or days to another; to determine staffing patterns including, but not limited to, the assignment of employees, number of employed, duties performed, qualifications required, and areas worked; to determine policies and procedures for patient care; to determine the equipment methods and procedures by which its operations are to be carried on; and to carry out the ordinary and customary functions of management subject only to such restrictions governing the exercise of these rights as are expressly specified in this agreement. The hospital has the unilateral right to determine all rules and regulations for the employees' working conditions, conduct, and health and safety. It has the sole right to eliminate and change all such rules and regulations.
>
> Nothing in this agreement shall be construed to limit or impair the right of the hospital to exercise its own discretion in determining whom to employ, and nothing in this agreement shall be interpreted as interfering in any way with the hospital's right to alter, rearrange or change, extend, limit, or curtail its operations or any part thereof; to decide upon the number of employees that may be assigned to work on any shift or the equipment to be employed in the performance of such work; or to shut down completely, whatever may be the effect upon employment, when in its sole discretion it may deem it advisable to do all or any of said things.

See *Kennecott Copper Corp.*, 148 NLRB 1653 (1964) for NLRB approval of the last paragraph supporting management's right to subcontract without having to bargain over the exercise of this right.

Protection of Union Activities. A contractual promise to avoid violating provisions already stipulated by the law gives the union "two bites of the apple." First, the union can take a claimed violation to arbitration. Even if the hospital secures a ruling in its favor, the union is still free to take the very same case to the NLRB. By its contractual promise, management has given the union an extra step.

Cost of Living Adjustment Clauses. The hospital that agrees to a cost of living adjustment (COLA) clause agrees to pay employees twice for the largest benefit that they receive.[11] One of the major components of the COLA figures is the cost of insurance premiums for health and welfare. Ordinarily, the employer has already agreed in the health and welfare insurance clause to pay increases in the insurance premiums for the term of the contract.

Pet Clauses of Management

Elimination of Past Practice. One clause that management should include in an agreement involves past practice. The clause should contain the following language:

> The union agrees and unqualifiedly waives its rights to bargain over any benefits not contained in this agreement and hereby recognizes and agrees that the hospital may discontinue any or all past practices not contained in this agreement and that this hospital may change any rules and regulations for its employees governing their conduct without bargaining with the union, whatever the effect may be upon employment.

Zipper Clause. In a zipper clause, the union agrees that it had a full and complete opportunity to discuss any and all of the clauses mentioned in the contract, as well as those clauses not mentioned, involving wages, hours, and working conditions. The union also specifically waives its right to bargain further over those conditions in this agreement.

BARGAINING TABLE GUIDELINES

It is imperative for the management team to follow these strategy guidelines:

1. At the inception of negotiations, take command of the bargaining table.
2. Do not allow the union to filibuster or intimidate the management team.
3. Be prepared to engage in dramatics to underscore a point.
4. Keep emotions under control.
5. Be sure that all language is clarified so that everyone understands the meaning of each word.
6. Submit a detailed proposal after reviewing the union's proposal. From that point forward, maneuver the union to work from the hospital's proposal, since the management team knows the intent of the hospital's proposed language.

7. Make only tentative agreements on pieces of the contract, and stipulate that, just as the union needs ratification of the agreements by its membership, the management team must have tentative agreements ratified by the board of directors when the contract is complete. Never indicate that the management team does not have the appropriate authority to act at the table.
8. Watch out for the language proposals, since they may be just as important as the economic proposals. For example, never allow the seniority clause to restrict management's right to transfer employees between jobs, shifts, or departments.
9. At the first negotiating session

   • review the entire union proposal for intent.
   • establish the union's authority to negotiate.
   • ask who comprises the union negotiating team and who their chief spokesperson will be; provide them with the same information.
   • attempt to secure the union's agreement to discuss and tentatively agree to all noneconomic items prior to discussing economics. Do not insist to impasse on this point, however.
   • tell the union that the management team will take detailed notes on all discussions, transcribe the notes, and provide written minutes to the union team. It is preferable to use management's notes as the record of the meetings rather than the union's notes.
   • set the time and frequency of regular bargaining sessions. Arrange meetings during normal work hours, but when the absence of the employees on the negotiating committee interferes least with business operations.
   • never hold any negotiating sessions on hospital premises, always select a neutral site so that the union negotiators cannot undermine the bargaining by immediately giving bits and pieces to the employees, which works to the political disadvantage of management.

10. In all stages of negotiations be sure to support management's positions with facts.
11. Never agree to open-ended retroactive pay; always have a deadline for securing the agreement. If there is no ending date, the union negotiator will have no incentive to end negotiations. Management may say, however, "The wage increase will be retroactive only if the complete contract with the wage increase is ratified by the membership in the next ten days."
12. Do not agree to an open-ended payment of the salaries of the union negotiating team, because to do so could establish a precedent requiring pay for all meetings on hospital time.

13. Furnish the union with all relevant information pertaining to the employees in the bargaining unit, i.e., names, wages, hours, working conditions, job descriptions, schedules, and seniority. Do not allow union negotiators access to employee personnel files, which are confidential and are the property of the hospital, although it may be necessary to show the union specific records within the file if they are relevant to the union's negotiating demands on health and safety or to specific disciplinary actions.
14. Sweep the office for surveillance devices, e.g., bugs, and place all important papers and proposals in locked file cabinets. Use a paper shredder to dispose of important papers that are discarded.

The nine cardinal rules that management must follow in collective bargaining negotiations are

1. Never agree to a clause that interferes with management's right to direct employees in their work assignments, such as a "mutual" consent clause that requires the employee's or the union's consent before an employee must perform an assigned task.
2. Never agree to a one-line management rights clause. Retained rights should be specifically delineated in order to minimize claims that management has waived certain rights. The employer will then have a better argument that the union has waived its right to bargain over such rights.
3. Never leave the negotiating table unilaterally. If the union is applying pressure, call a caucus and work out the time and conditions for attending the next session.
4. Never allow the union to accuse management of bad faith bargaining without setting the record straight *immediately* on the factual situation supporting good faith bargaining.
5. Never tell a third party, such as a federal or state mediator, anything about management's bargaining strategy or positions that should not be told to the union at the table.
6. Never fail to inform all managers immediately after the session has ended what happened at the table and what they may say to employees about respective employees and events.
7. Never tell employees what has not been discussed at the table. In the same vein, do not send a letter to the employees until management has made its last and final offer, and has firmly decided what to do if the union and the membership reject the offer.
8. Never say that the hospital cannot grant the union's demands on wages because of its "inability" to pay. If the hospital does so plead, the union may examine the hospital's books. (See *NLRB v Truitt Mfg. Co.,* 351 U.S. 149 [1956]). Instead, the way to avoid the union's looking at your books is for

the hospital to refuse to grant the union's demands on wages by stating that to do so would make the hospital noncompetitive.
9. Never say "never."

LABOR CONTRACTS IN HOSPITALS

Collective bargaining is relatively new to the health care industry. In a study of labor agreements in 6,199 hospitals, it was concluded that, as hospitals become more seasoned in union matters, labor contracts in hospitals will become similar to those in other industries.[12] Even early in the 1970s, hospital contracts contained language that was surprisingly like that in the contracts of other industries. Contract duration was shorter, and clauses on wage reopeners were more common in the hospital industry, however. Union shop clauses were included significantly less often than in other types of businesses. Dues checkoff clauses and statements prohibiting discrimination against those involved in union activities were more common. Because of the licensure and occupational restrictions inherent in the hospital, there were differences in relation to seniority; these clauses frequently included some reference to transfer policies. The area of discipline and grievance/arbitration procedures were stressed in these hospital contracts as much as in those of other types of businesses.

While this study showed that the issues of layoff, recall, severance, subcontracting, and worker group size were not as critical in hospital contracts as in other industrial contracts, recent contracts suggest that more emphasis will be placed on these items in the 1980s because of such factors as inflation, unemployment, cost constraints, and multihospital corporation acquisitions. The emphasis in the contracts studied on wage-related provisions, such as shift differential, premium pay for weekends and holidays, on-call pay, and unscheduled call-back pay, will probably continue in the 1980s. In the contracts studied, the number of holidays and holiday pay for those who work were behind those in general industry, however, when holiday time is supplemented with sick time figures, the hospital industry was well on its way to a four-day week.

In a few cases, when the hospitals negotiated with professionals in a bargaining unit, continuing education orientation and some unit involvement in decision making were emphasized.[13] In the 1980s, a continuing issue in professional labor contracts in hospitals will be practice and delivery of health care services; under the legal constraints such as TEFRA, which has resulted in DRGs. Contracts already include items such as the American Nurses' Association code, provisions for joint practice committees, patient ratios as computed from patient classification systems, language on work assignments, and job security.[14]

A very recent trend is the hospital's elimination of participation in the Social Security system. However, this is a mandatory subject of bargaining.

The management negotiating team should study the specific positions taken by the group involved. For example, if nurses' associations are involved, they might study the nursing literature, e.g., *The American Nurse*, the publications of the American Nurses' Association, and the *American Journal of Nursing*. The news section in the *American Journal of Nursing* often provides current material on issues and what is happening on the union scene. To get a perspective on women in hospitals and unions from the *union's* perspective, the management team should read *The New Nightingales: Hospital Workers, Unions, New Women's Issues* by Patricia Cayo Sexton.[15] Above all, they should remember that a part of being successful in an adversary relationship is knowing the opponent.

SUCCESSORSHIP

Hospitals that are making acquisitions or are themselves being acquired should study the effect of successorship on labor relations. In order to be bound to the union, a successor must hire a majority of the predecessor's employees represented by that union. A successor cannot refuse to hire these employees, however, solely to avoid recognizing the union.

If there is a union contract in effect, a successor is not required to assume that agreement, as held by the U.S. Supreme Court in *NLRB v. Burns International Security Services, Inc.*, 92 S.Ct. 1571 (1972). In order to avoid doing so, however, the successor must not take over the hospital without informing the union and the employees involved that employees will be hired only on the successor's terms and conditions, which differ from those stated in the union contract. If the employees hired on these terms and conditions form a majority of the old bargaining unit, a new agreement must be negotiated with the unit.[16] The successor who wants the existing agreement simply takes over the hospital "as is," hiring the same employees with the same wages, hours, and working conditions.

NOTES

1. Bureau of National Affairs, *Basic Patterns in Union Contracts* (Washington, DC: Bureau of National Affairs, 1979).

2. Hervey A. Juris, "Collective Bargaining in Hospitals: Labor Agreements in the Hospital Industry," *Labor Law Journal* 28 (August 1977):504—511.

3. Bureau of National Affairs, "Employee Benefits in Medium and Large Firms," *Daily Labor Report,* 24 September 1982: E-1.

4. Benjamin Taylor and Fred Witney, *Labor Relations Law,* 4th ed. (Englewood Cliffs, NJ: Prentice-Hall, 1983).

5. Available from Bureau of Labor Statistics, Department of Labor, Washington, DC 20210.

6. Bureau of National Affairs, *Basic Patterns.*

7. "Characteristics of Major Collective Bargaining Agreements," Bulletin 2065 (Washington, DC: Bureau of Labor Statistics, U.S. Department of Labor, April 1980).

8. Ibid.

9. Juris, "Collective Bargaining in Hospitals."

10. Suzanne LaViolette, "Job Security Hot Subject for Unions," *Modern Healthcare* 12 (August 1982):33–34.

11. Clarence R. Deitsch and David A. Dilts, "The COLA Clause: An Employer Bargaining Weapon?" *Personnel Journal* 59 (March 1982):220–223.

12. Hervey A. Juris, *Labor Agreements in the Hospital Industry: A Study of Collective Bargaining Outputs* (Sponsored by the National Center for Health Services Research and the American Hospital Association under Grant No. 5 R18HS 01577–02).

13. Juris, "Collective Bargaining in Hospitals."

14. LaViolette, "Job Security."

15. Patricia Cayo Sexton, *The New Nightingales: Hospital Workers, Unions, New Women's Issues* (New York: Enquiry Press, 1982).

16. Norman Metzger, "Labor Relations Demand Special Attention in Multihospital Systems," *Hospitals* 55 (January 1981):57–59.

Chapter 5

Strikes

Strikes have become increasingly more frequent over the past few years. The first recorded work stoppage occurred in 1937 when Local 171 of the Hospital Employees Association staged a kitchen sit-in at Jewish Hospital of Brooklyn to protest low wages, poor working conditions, and the discharge of a fellow employee. Most recent hospital strikes have involved nurses and physicians rather than nonprofessional workers. In 1981, Aliqueppa Hospital in Aliqueppa, Pennsylvania reduced its census of 175 to 7 because of a District 1199 strike involving housekeeping, maintenance, dietary, and nursing personnel. In 1981, when Local 1199 struck Highlands Regional Medical Center in Prestonburg, Kentucky, the fifteen-week job action resulted in violence.

Over the past decade the state nurses' associations have been involved in numerous strikes. The American Nurses' Association (ANA) has widely espoused its belief that it alone can solve the unique problems of the nursing profession. When faced with a strike at its Kansas City headquarters in 1978, however, the ANA reacted more like an employer than a labor organization and advertised for striker replacements in a local newspaper.

Nurses have shown repeatedly that they are willing to strike to gain desired concessions from hospital administrations. Certainly, unique issues of patient care standards, ethics, and staffing around the clock in health care institutions create a specialized type of labor problem in nursing. Settling these problems in nursing is a top priority for hospital managers, since nurses comprise the largest group of employees in a hospital. When nurses walk out, hospitals must either restrict services drastically or close completely. For example, in 1981 nurses staged a seventeen-day strike at Cape Cod Hospital in Hyannis, Massachusetts for wages and benefits that caused the hospital to shut down all patient services except the emergency room. A strike by other categories of workers has a less drastic effect on hospital operations.

Strikes are also getting longer and more intense. The strike at Berkshire Medical Center in Pittsfield, Massachusetts lasted sixty-nine days. In 1981, a two-month strike closed the hospital in Hibbins, Minnesota. Springfield, Oregon was the site of an eighty-four day strike in the summer of 1981. The longest strike involving nurses occurred in Ashtabula, Ohio where strikers were active for nearly sixteen months.

ETHICAL IMPLICATIONS

The power to strike is the most dangerous weapon of the union. Health care workers strike when they believe that their needs and concerns are being ignored, but they are often disturbed by the increased suffering and possible permanent damage or death that their right to protest worker wages and working conditions causes patients. Unions justify the patient suffering and death by stating that a strike can do a greater good for humanity in the long run.

Managers must realize that employees are more educated than ever before and that they have high expectations in career, employment rewards, and quality of life. Thus, they are reevaluating their jobs in terms of the short- and long-term picture. Managers must let employees know that they are interested in primary intervention in employee problems; managers must emphasize that (1) they can be trusted, (2) they are sensitive to employee needs, (3) they believe in contemporary management techniques that emphasize "the people skills," (4) they are willing to include employees in decision making, and (5) strikes do not settle problems—only hard work and committed collaborative effort do.

UNION PROPAGANDA AND MANAGEMENT RESPONSES

1. Professional employees must control the number and kind of staff and what they do so that administrators will operate the hospital properly.
2. Strikes are the only way to force administrators to give priority to nursing causes and demands. Without strikes, administrators are complacent and unconcerned.
3. Withdrawing nursing care is no more unethical than continuing care under poor conditions.
4. The public needs to know how unsafe nursing care is in this hospital.
5. Improved wages, benefits, and working conditions make happier health care workers, and these satisfied workers will give better care to future patients. The short-term compromises in patient care are worth it.
6. Strikes result in better conditions and make the hospital more attractive to qualified professionals.

7. Nurses have a contract with the institution. Striking breaks no contract with patients, because there is none.
8. Nurses are not responsible for unforeseen deaths and injuries arising from a strike, these are unintended consequences.

The preceding eight statements represent some of the major arguments that unions make when they are trying to persuade nurses to strike. There are a number of actions managers can take to counter the statements of the union:

- Build a trusting relationship with employees. Managers should let employees know that management can be counted on for daily needs and for long-term needs. It is easy for employees who mistrust managers to unionize and strike.
- Revamp the administration into one that communicates closely and frequently with employees; know the issues, needs, and concerns of both individuals and employee groups.
- Educate managers on labor relations.
- Broadcast the rationale for remaining union-free.
- Publicize the hospital's commitment to high-quality patient care and to its employees; respond to employee input, concerns, and needs.
- Show employees that there is no positive correlation between increased rewards and improved patient care, if the union raises the question.
- Ask how an economic strike guarantees improved patient care and who really benefits—the employee or the patient.
- Make employees accountable. If they want to strike, they must take responsibility for endangering the lives of citizens, friends, and families. They are morally responsible for what happens, because their prior knowledge of these consequences makes them voluntarily responsible.
- Bring criminal charges against individuals who may have violated the law in a moment of peaked emotion.
- Point out that strikes undermine patient care and contradict their own reasons for entering the health care field.
- Reinforce reality. The problems in the health care professions did not develop overnight and cannot be resolved overnight. Resolution is something that will take time, energy, and input from all involved parties. Other issues are beyond the control of the hospital, since the hospital is bound by mandates from governmental agencies and accrediting bodies.
- Keep employees informed about real issues. Many times the reason for a strike is not what employees think it is. Instead, the strike may be politically motivated. Sometimes a union calls a strike over seemingly noble issues just to remind the employees that it is looking out for employee interests.

- Emphasize that the professional roles of employees have continued to improve in recent years in regard to expansion of and improvement in the role and support systems of the nurse in patient care.

There are many reasons for a strike. Economic issues can be a major reason; improvement of patient care standards is a nobler cause. The real reason often has more to do with politics and power struggles between the union and the employer, however. Strikes are easier to sell in areas where unions are strong in surrounding industries and strikes are an accepted way of life for families and friends of employees. Nurses who are caught up in the women's rights movement often believe that the strike is for independent input in decision making, improved self-worth and status, and their inherent rights as human beings. Whole workshops are given to union organizers on how to use the women's rights movement as a technique to convince women to organize and to strike.[1]

LAWFUL STRIKES

The Health Care Amendments to the National Labor Relations Act (NLRA) made special provisions for strikes in health care institutions. When the parties are unable to resolve their problems, the party who provided the original notice of the dispute must also notify the Federal Mediation and Conciliation Service (FMCS), which may appoint a board of inquiry to investigate the dispute, stipulate the facts discovered, and write recommendations that are not binding to the involved parties. When no settlement is reached and the mandatory time periods have lapsed, the union may strike after it has provided the FMCS and the employer with a ten-day notice.

The Mediation Process

A required alternative to a strike in a health care facility is mediation. In the mediation process, a neutral third party acts as a catalyst to facilitate negotiations between the two parties. The mediator does not make decisions or substantiate content of any resolutions, a fact that distinguishes mediators from arbitrators.[2]

The work of the FMCS is done by more than 300 commissioners from about eighty major cities. To qualify as a mediator, the candidate must have seven years of direct experience at the bargaining table and must be appointed by the FMCS. The director of the FMCS is selected by the President. In order to understand the personal biases that the mediator brings to the situation, hospital administrators should know the type of experience that a mediator with whom they are dealing has had.

While a mediator may be asked to work with labor and management on disputes or concerns at any time during the term of the contract, a mediator's presence in disputes that could result in a strike is mandated by the Health Care Amendments. The mediator must be well acquainted with health care to participate in all the formal and off-the-record meetings required to bring labor and management together. Only a well-versed mediator can ask the in-depth questions that reveal the unique issues of health care, the implications of union activity and a strike against a health care institution, and the contemporary conditions affecting the attitudes and well-being of health care workers.

Sometimes, despite the mediator's attempt and the work of the board of inquiry, no settlement is reached between labor and management. In such cases, the union provides the FMCS and the employer with a ten-day notice of a strike. During this ten-day period and during the strike itself, mediation continues. The mediator remains involved until the strike is resolved. This involvement extends to include a role as an educator and as an advisor in human relations, as well as the traditional role of a go-between.[3-5]

Interpretation of the Ten-Day Notice

It is an unfair labor practice for a hospital to try to circumvent the collective bargaining process by using ten-day notice period to stockpile supplies or to hire replacements for those who might strike. Likewise, it is an unfair labor practice for the union to harass the employer by continually giving strike notices without following through with the job action.

In the case of *District 1199 v. Parkway Pavillion Healthcare,* 222 NLRB No. 15 (1976), enforcement denied, 82LC ¶ 10,042 (CA2, 1976) the National Labor Relations Board (NLRB) stipulated guidelines for interpreting Section 8(g) of the NLRA as follows:

1. It is mandatory for labor organizations to give written notice of a strike to the employer and the FMCS.
2. The notice requirement is not affected by the rationale for picketing.
3. There is no language in Section 8(g) that modifies the provision on a circumstantial basis.

Even a sympathy strike of a second union is a violation of Section 8(g) if the second union has not filed its own ten-day notice on striking. For example, in *Hospital and Institutional Workers' Union, Local 250, SEIU, AFL-CIO and Affiliated Hospitals of San Francisco et al.,* 255 NLRB No. 81 (1981), a unit of cooks from several health care institutions sent to the FMCS and the multiemployer association a strike notice that did not specify the date and time when the strike would start. While a second notice with all of the facts was sent to the employer, the union not only failed to send a second notice to the FMCS, but also commenced the strike less than ten days after the association's receipt of the second notice. Local 250 did not file the requisite notice, but it joined Local 2, the cooks, in a sympathy strike, even though the original strike was unlawful. The NLRB affirmed the administrative law judge's finding that Local 250 was in violation of Section 8(g) of the NLRA.

NLRB actions over the past few years have convinced labor law specialists in health care that each instance of picketing or work stoppage at a health care facility is carefully and individually analyzed to determine if Section 8(g) of the NLRA has been violated. Managers should realize that Section 8(g) applies only to labor unions, however, not to employees who are unorganized. Thus, concerted activity by employees is protected. Several cases illustrate the point that a walkout by employees is not in violation of the NLRA when a labor organization is not orchestrating the job action, e.g., *Long Beach Youth Center v. NLRB*, 591 F.2d 1276 (9th Cir. 1979); *NLRB v. Rock Hill Convalescent Center*, 585 F.2d 700 (4th Cir. 1978); *Vil Care*, 249 NLRB No. 95 (1980); *Walker Methodist Residence and Health Care, Inc.*, 227 NLRB No. 238 (1977).

The ten-day notice requirement is not applicable to instances of protected concerted activity, as shown by the case of *East Chicago Rehabilitation Center, Inc. v. NLRB* (CA-7) 710 F.2d 397 (1983). In this case, the Seventh Circuit Court of Appeals enforced an NLRB decision (259 NLRB No. 135) that, even though employees staged a two-hour strike without giving the ten-day notice required by Section 8(g) of the NLRA, their protest was still "protected concerted activity." Seventeen health care workers had staged a spontaneous two-hour walkout in protest of their employer's unilateral act of forbidding employees to eat lunch away from the center's premises. Even though some of the center's routines were disrupted by the walkout of less than half of the day shift employees for a two-hour period, there was no evidence that patient safety or health had been jeopardized. In a lengthy dissent, Judge John Coffey of the Seventh Circuit rebuked the majority for setting a dangerous precedent of treating the health care workers as though they were workers on an assembly line, in a steel mill, or in a coal mine, where walking off the job without notice would cause at most an interruption in production. Judge Coffey stated: "I dissent as I believe it is important to emphasize that this walkout occurred in the health care field, where human lives are all too frequently hanging in the balance."

In *East Chicago Rehabilitation Center,* the union had no prior notice of the walkout, did not authorize it, and, therefore, did not have to give the ten-day notice required by Section 8(g) of the NLRA. Nor did the employees use the walkout to replace the union as their bargaining representative. The Seventh Circuit stated that neither Section 9(a), which makes the union the exclusive bargaining representative, nor Section 8(g), which imposes a ten-day notice requirement on strikes in health care institutions, removed the protection afforded by Section 7. The employer was found to be in violation of Sections 8(a)(1) and 8(g) of the NLRA in unlawfully discharging employees for engaging in a protected strike, and the center was ordered to reinstate the strikers with back pay.

A contractor that is doing work at a health care institution and becomes involved in a strike does not have to comply with Section 8(g) unless the job action involves employees of the health care institution.

In another type of case involving the ten-day strike notice the union was found to be operating in good faith. In *Southwest Louisiana Hospital Association (Lake Charles Memorial Hospital) v. Office and Professional Employees Local 87*, 664 F.2d 1321 (1982), the union filed a strike notice that complied with Section 213 of the LMRA. The hospital filed suit in federal district court against the union claiming that since a fact finder was properly appointed, the union was bound to maintain the status quo under Section 213 of the LMRA, as amended, and by its giving a strike notice during the status quo, it breached the status quo thus forcing the hospital to prepare for the strike and to incur damages. The damages the hospital claimed included purchasing concrete blocks to protect the hospital's vital supplies; installing an eight-foot-high chain link fence around the rear of the hospital; increasing the security personnel; and, decreasing the number of non-emergency patient admissions.

However, the court found that the FMCS did not appoint a fact finder or board of inquiry within the time limits provided by Section 213 of the LMRA governing establishment of boards of inquiry, and the union's two strike notices neither breached any contract nor violated Section 213 of the LMRA —specifically that provision requiring the maintaining of the status quo for 15 days after a fact finder is appointed or a board of inquiry is established.

A significant point in this case is that the court cited, with apparent approval, the district court's finding that a strike notice alone does not breach the status quo under Section 213, on the theory that Section 213 fails to specifically prohibit threats to strike. The court then cites *District 1199-E, National Union of Hospital and Health Care Employees*, 227 NLRB No. 132 (1976), to the effect that a threat to strike does not breach Section 8(d) because that section, unlike other NLRA sections, does not specifically prohibit threats.

Further, the constitutionality of Section 8(g) has been challenged as an infringement of free speech rights guaranteed under the First Amendment in *District 1199 RWDSU (United Hospitals of Newark)*, 232 NLRB No. 67 (1977). The Board held that a "demonstration" at a hospital constituted picketing, even though no work stoppage resulted and, as such, was banned by Section 8(g), which prohibits all forms of picketing without the proper 10-day notice. The Board further held that the 10-day notice requirement was not an abridgment of freedom of speech.

The validity of Section 8(g) has also been tested when it was at variance with a state statute. In *New York v. Hotel, Nursing Home and Allied Health Services*

Union, 410 F.Supp. 225 (D.C. N.Y. 1976), the court ruled that federal law preempts state statutes.

Injunctive Relief

When the Norris-LaGuardia Act was initially passed, it deprived the federal courts of the power to issue injunctions in certain labor disputes, under Sections 4 and 7, unless certain procedural prerequisites were met. The decision in *The Boys Markets, Inc. v. Retail Clerks Local 770,* 398 U.S. 235 (1970), created a narrow exception to Norris-LaGuardia. When a contract with a no-strike and no-lockout clause and a mandatory provision for arbitration on grievances, is in effect, the union may not strike and management may not lock employees out. If either party violates the contract *over an arbitrable dispute,* a *Boys Market* injunction may be issued and the party in violation of the contract may be compelled to take its grievance to arbitration.

Another famous case in the area of injunctive relief is *Buffalo Forge Co. v. United Steelworkers of America AFL-CIO,* 96 S.Ct. 3141 (1976). In this case, the Supreme Court refused to grant injunctive relief in sympathy strike situations. The Court reasoned that it could not grant such relief as a sympathy strike, by its very nature, is not over an arbitrable dispute—one of the main conditions for an injunction the Supreme Court required in the *Boys Markets* case.

While these cases are landmark cases in labor law, experts believe that cases specific to health care labor law will be heard in response to the special needs of the industry. For example, in *Alsup v. Drug and Hospital Union 1199,* 91 LRRM 2063 (DC NY 1975), an employer discharged a union member for participating in a wildcat strike. The employee appealed his case to arbitration while the employer made a motion for an injunction, claiming that since the discharge involved alleged violations of the NLRA, the matter should be resolved by the NLRB and not by an arbitrator. The district court held that, although this was a matter arguably involving an unfair labor practice, the case may be hard in arbitration proceedings, because the primary purpose of the NLRA is to encourage settlement of disputes through arbitration.

In the Health Care Amendments Section 8(d) was modified to read: "Any employee who engages in any strike within the appropriate period specified in subsection (g) of this Section shall lose his status as an employee." While not the same as losing the job, the loss of protected status as an employee removes the individual from coverage under the NLRA.

TYPES OF STRIKES

There are several types of strikes: (a) an organizational strike, (b) a strike alleging that the employer has committed unfair labor practices, (c) an economic strike resulting from disagreements in negotiations, (d) a wildcat strike, and (e) secondary boycott strikes.

During the periods in which the NLRA bars strikes, a strike of any kind is illegal, and involved strikers are not entitled to reinstatement into their jobs. Strikers who violate a no-strike agreement in a contract lose the protection of their employee status under the NLRA. Finally, strikers who commit unlawful acts as a part of the strike not only lose their employee status protection under the NLRA, but also can be lawfully discharged by the hospital. For example, strikers can be discharged for serious picket line misconduct.

Concerning picket line misconduct, it is interesting to note a recent detailed four-year study completed on picket line violence. The findings are contained in a 540-page report titled, "Union Violence: The Record and the Response by Courts, Legislatures, and the NLRB," published by The Wharton School of the University of Pennsylvania. This report documents the fact that federal and state courts, as well as the NLRB, have been "soft" and have "coddled" strikers who are guilty of violent crimes during the strikes. According to the authors, professor of law Thomas R. Haggard of the University of South Carolina and associate professor of management Armand J. Thieblot of the University of Maryland, numerous decisions by state and federal courts and by the NLRB reveal a high degree of tolerance for strike-related violence and conduct that would clearly be a criminal violation under normal circumstances, when it occurs in the context of a strike, becomes what the NLRB calls "animal exuberance," not to be condoned but not to be taken seriously either.

A very interesting finding identifies the United Mine Workers Union and the Teamsters Union as the "worst offenders" when it comes to union violence, based on an analysis of the thousands of cases the professors reviewed. The report also states that a review of violence-related cases heard by the NLRB shows "repeated appearances" by unions representing construction workers, meatcutters, machinists, and, "in recent years," health care workers. The information for the report was further supported by a list of 2,598 incidents of violence involving these unions drawn from newspaper reports between 1975 and 1981. A summary of this report can be found in the Bureau of National Affairs' *Daily Labor Report*, No. 164, at page A-8, dated August 23, 1983.

Organizational Strike

In an organizational strike, the union strikes when the employer refuses to recognize the union without an election. By calling a strike, the union hopes to force the employer to recognize the union in its organizing drive. The union does not normally organize this way, and in this type of strike, employees that are striking may be permanently replaced.

Unfair Labor Practice Strike

A union may call a strike to protest the hospital's alleged unfair labor practices, saying that such unfair labor practices interfere with the rights of employees. When the strike is over, the hospital may be required to reinstate striking employees with their full rights and privileges if it is held to have committed the alleged unfair labor practices. This means that, if the employer has hired replacements, the strikers have first choice on reinstatement, and their replacements must be discharged or moved to other positions.

Economic Strike

It is to the hospital's advantage to prove that the employees are engaged in an economic strike, because an employer can permanently replace strikers in an economic strike. This area of law is complex, however. A striker cannot be discharged for participating in an economic strike, only replaced. Before deciding to go the route of permanently replacing strikers in an economic strike, the employer should be aware that it is a long-term, expensive, difficult ordeal to go through all the problems and litigation involved in the process. This is particularly true in light of the recent U.S. Supreme Court decision in *Belknap, Inc. v. Hale,* (1983, U.S.) 103 S.Ct. 3172, 113 LRRM 3057, which held that when an employer exercises its legal right to hire replacements and promises them "permanent" positions, it cannot then fire them to take back the strikers, even if done through agreement with the union. The Court held that if the replacements are fired to take back the strikers, the substitutes have a valid action in state court to sue for breach of contract and misrepresentation.

A strike that, at its inception, is an economic one may be converted into an unfair practice strike if the employer commits violations of the law that prolong the strike. This can occur, for example, if the employer engages in surface bargaining (i.e., merely going through the motions without any intent to reach an agreement), has a "take it or leave it" attitude at the table, or submits proposals that take away any voice the union might have in representing the employees.

Wildcat Strike

Strikes or partial strikes staged by employees without the approval of their union are wildcat strikes. Such strikes typically occur when there is a no-strike and no-lockout clause in the contract and union members believe that they have suffered an injustice either because their union is not adequately representing them or because the hospital is ignoring the grievance procedure provided by contract. Wildcat strikers are protected for their action only when they take such action because the employer has committed serious NLRA violations that undermine the union, as set out in *Mastro Plastic Corporation v. NLRB* 350 U.S. 270 (1956).

It is wise for the hospital to insist on a provision in the contract whereby in the event of strikes unauthorized by the union, the union's officers must comply with the following steps:

1. The union agrees to notify the hospital and the employees that such action is not authorized within 12 hours of the job action.
2. The union will work cooperatively with the hospital. All union officials will report for work as an example to the striking employees and will do everything within their power to end or avoid the strike.
3. The union recognizes the rights of the employer to discipline any employees engaged in such activities, up to and including discharge, which degree of discipline will not be an issue in arbitration, and that the arbitrator will only decide whether the involved employee participated in the unauthorized work stoppage.

In a recent Supreme Court case, *Bowen v. American Postal Workers' Union*, 103 S.Ct. 588 (1983, U.S.), the high court ruled in a 5 to 4 decision that the union was liable for a part of the wages that an employee had lost because of his unlawful discharge. In their opinion, the Justices found that the union had breached its duty of fair representation and had to bear its responsibility for its failure to take the matter to arbitration. In the opinion, Justice Lewis F. Powell, Jr. stated. "There is no unfairness to the union in this approach. . . . By seeking and acquiring the exclusive right and power to speak for a group of employees, the union assumes a corresponding duty to discharge that responsibility faithfully." *Bowen* could affect contract negotiations in many areas, as the employer can legally ask for union indemnification in those areas in which the union is asking for joint rights (i.e., joint rights result in joint responsibility). Also, this decision could have a bearing on wildcat strikes that are attributed to a lack of fair representation by the union, namely, where employers are able, to sue the union for monetary damages caused by the strike.

Secondary Boycott Strike

Section 8(b)(4) of the NLRA addresses the issue of a secondary boycott. In this instance, because of a dispute with Hospital A, the union causes other companies or health care agencies to avoid doing business with Hospital A. The *primary* employer is Hospital A, and the *secondary* employer is the business or health care agency that the union is urging to boycott Hospital A. The secondary employer is frequently a customer or supplier of the primary employer. For example, if Hospital A refuses to recognize it, the union pickets at the site of the hospital's laundry service so that it will stop doing business with Hospital A. This is an illegal secondary boycott.

In general, Section 8(b)(4) prohibits secondary boycotts and the threat of them. Section 8(b)(4)(B) does not, however, protect the secondary employer who is on Hospital A's premises from incidental action arising from the picketing of the primary employer; it is lawful for the union at Hospital A, for example, to ask laundry employees of the secondary employer not to cross the picket line at Hospital A. It is also lawful under the proper management rights clause for an employer to subcontract work that is normally done by the primary employer's employees. However, when a secondary employer abandons neutral status and becomes an ally in the dispute between the union and Hospital A, the secondary employer becomes a primary employer and is not protected from secondary boycotts and strikes.

When a primary and secondary employer occupy the same premises, the union striking the primary employer may not direct action against secondary employers on the same site. The standard for lawful picketing against a primary employer was determined in a case known as *Moore Dry Dock,* 81 NLRB 1108 (1949). As long as the objective of the picketing is not unlawful, separate gates are often established for workers uninvolved in the job action so that picketing can be confined to the primary employer.

Steps To Take When the Picket Arrives

When a contractor, e.g., a construction company or its subcontractors, have pickets at a hospital site, the hospital and/or contractor should take the following steps:

1. Clearly mark entrances or gates to be used by the struck contractor, its employees, and its suppliers. Mark entrance(s) clearly for employees. Do not deviate from the entrance requirements of each gate.
2. Locate the gate for picketers as far away as possible from hospital entrances and delivery gates/entrances where hospital supplies are delivered.
3. Fence the picketed area to emphasize the need to use only designated entrances.
4. Make gate signs sturdy, legible, and large enough to be read from a truck driver's seat. Sign should read: This gate to be used by *only* (list contractors, their employees, and their suppliers). All others must use different gate.
5. Meet with contractors to establish procedure for gates and picketing, as well as special considerations for health care institutions.
6. Obtain the name, address, and telephone number of each union business agent whose union could picket at the site.

7. Familiarize managers with what to do in cases of violence.
8. Hire a security guard for each entrance to monitor access of only specified people. Try to get the contractor to pay for the security guard at each entrance.
9. Give security guards a stop sign, a clipboard with forms to report any incidents, and permission to ask for identification of anyone entering the gate/entrance.
10. Copy the words on the picketers' signs. Note the number of pickets, the date and time of their arrival, and the location of picketing. *Very important:* Ask the picketers to explain the purpose of their picketing. Report all this information to the hospital's labor attorney.
11. Send a telegram to the picketing union notifying them that separate gates are being established.
12. If a picketer does not honor the separate gates, send a telegram to the union agent and call the agent. If you get no results, notify the NLRB.
13. Work with your labor attorney closely to protect your legal position, as picketing is intricate legally.

STRIKE PLANNING

Even though the union is required to provide notice of strikes, administrators should not wait until then to formulate a strike plan. Soon after the union has been recognized, a strike management committee should be formed; it should be composed of key people, such as the chief of staff, personnel director, legal counsel, purchasing department head, accountant, administrator for hospital operations, security chief, and the administrator for nursing services. The director of public relations is a likely candidate for the strike management committee, since that individual often handles news releases to the media. The committee should be no larger than twelve people, and these individuals must be committed to management.

Each committee member should be assigned specific areas of responsibility to ensure that all critical services of the hospital are covered. After receiving the assignment, each committee member should prepare a contingency plan that can be implemented either for continuing operations or for shutting down the hospital, either partially or totally. For example, the security department should map out all entrances, fences, and windows that would need to be secured and should plan for security in parking lots, employee entrances, and patient entrances. The legal department should prepare injunction pleadings that can be quickly individualized to the situation and filed.

The labor relations department should inform all departments of the contract expiration date, the status of negotiations, and the implications of these events as they relate to a strike. The labor relations department should also begin educational sessions with all managers to inform them about strikes in general and possible employer responses. Specific facts of the strike contingency plan should not be revealed to the group as a whole until later, however.

The personnel department should prepare contingency plans for advertising for and hiring replacements, utilizing personnel, laying off nonstrikers in case of a hospital shutdown, and distributing wages and benefits. A list of companies and agencies that need official notification in the event of a strike should be compiled.

The purchasing and accounting departments should arrange for the use of alternate suppliers and establish a master list for notification of vendors and suppliers. They also need to investigate the possibility of renting a public warehouse to which supplies can be delivered. Hospital or non-union truck drivers can then pick up these supplies. Such arrangements are necessary, because unions that honor the picket line will prevent truck drivers from delivering vital supplies and equipment to the hospital.

The nursing director and medical director must plan to continue safe care for patients. This includes planning to use emergency vehicles and the facilities of other health care institutions, when necessary. Certain units can be closed, surgery and other services can be limited, and special staffing schedules can be implemented. The plan should include room and board arrangements for nurses, inhalation therapists, laboratory technicians, dietary personnel, radiology technicians, and other key personnel who may be unable to leave the hospital at times.[6]

The chief operating officer should direct the total plan and may be the logical choice for coordinating the communications network. During this preplanning stage, this executive must see that all the needs of the hospital have been considered.

At this time, the chief executive officer can address the managerial group and provide them with the hospital's philosophy on coping with strikes, managing in a union environment, and continuing operations in the event of a strike. The administrator should offer to answer questions and should indicate who the chief communications person will be during the strike. The exact mechanism for clearing all information through that person should be stipulated. Managers may be given some prepared questions and answers to learn so that they may respond to employee questions. These questions should be updated periodically so that they are relevant to current issues.

Taking a Strike

When a contract is being negotiated, management must set limits on the compromises that the hospital can make with the union. Hospitals that believe they cannot stand a strike may give so many concessions that, in the long run, the concessions become more expensive than a strike would be. When managers decide on a hospital's ability to weather a strike, they must answer the following questions:

- What are the strike issues? For example, would the union strike to get a union shop? Would the hospital take one over this issue?
- How do hospital wages, benefits, and working conditions compare to area and industry standards?
- Is the hospital in a position to take a strike?
- Considering all factors, how long could the hospital survive under strike conditions?
- What type of personnel is available in the area if the strikers need to be permanently replaced?
- Which union demands can the hospital accept, and which demands must the hospital reject?
- How will the community, e.g., health care providers, competing hospitals, the public, and the employees, react to the strike?
- Can the hospital obtain the necessary supplies, staff, and equipment to function safely during a strike?
- What instructions will be given to managers?
- What is the hospital's labor relations history? How would a strike affect all involved parties?
- Do the union negotiators control the membership?
- What percentage of the hospital's employees would go out on the strike?
- Does the union have strike benefits? If so, how much does it have in reserve, and when would strike benefits begin for strikers?
- Are strikers eligible for unemployment compensation, food stamps, or welfare in the state?
- Would other unions respect the picket line or join in a sympathy strike?
- What are the hospital's chances of achieving its objectives in a strike?
- How strong is the union, and how long are its members prepared to strike?
- How long can strikers hold out when their living expenses are continuing?

WHEN A STRIKE IS INEVITABLE

Management should take the following steps when a strike is inevitable:

1. Implement the strike plan that has been preplanned, after adjusting it to the realities of the actual situation.

2. Formalize the strike management committee, and ask them to put their plans into operation.
3. Inform all department heads of the reasons for the strike, give them the information they need, and review assigned roles and responsibilities.
4. Set up the communication network.
5. Establish a strike log (Exhibit 5-1) and an operations center.
6. Designate the person who will keep a complete record of all strike incidents (Exhibit 5-2), including statements from victims and witnesses of these incidents (Exhibit 5-3).
7. Designate the spokesperson for the hospital.
8. Warn managers not to speak to union members concerning negotiations on the picket line unless a representative of the hospital is present.

Management must review its contingency plan for continued operations or for an orderly shutdown. If the hospital continues to operate, management must pay employees whatever the contract guarantees them up to the day the strike begins. Employees should be informed by mail that they may maintain health and welfare

---

Exhibit 5–1 Sample Strike Log

> Record in chronological order incidents at your assigned gate. Use brief notations with emphasis on critical detail—the who, what, when, where, and how of events as they occur.

Normally prepared by: (Observer witnessing events)
Normal routing: (Supervisor)

_____   _____   _____

Gate Number   Date   Observer's name (print)

Time	Incident

Exhibit 5–2 Sample Strike Incident Report

```
Person witnessing incident _____
                                        (please print)
Department _____Supervisor's name _____
Telephone number _____
Date and time                          Location where
incident observed _____  incident occurred _____


                    Brief Description of Incident

_____

_____

_____

_____

_____


    Note: Brief description of incident should include identification of victim and offender, if any:
other persons present at the time of incident who may have witnessed it and any other pertinent
details.


                                 _____
                                           Signed

                                 _____
                                            Date
```

insurance during the strike only by making individual arrangements to assume the total payment of premiums for said plans during the strike with the personnel director. Individual contact with the employee is preferable, because the personnel director can obtain important feedback for management.

The personnel department should prepare a master list of all employees, complete with their addresses, telephone numbers, and pictures, if possible. A set of envelopes should be addressed to all employees and held ready for the time when an expedited mailing is needed. Once the strike begins, a list of strikers and nonstrikers should be prepared. It is important for management to maintain duplicate copies of all important documents in a safe place.

When the issue of hiring permanent replacements arises, management should write a letter to employees (Exhibit 5-4) before the actual hiring takes place. The public relations department should prepare various news releases, such as the one in Exhibit 5-5. Management also should prepare and distribute instructions to employees early in the strike process so that employees know what to do when they come to work (Exhibit 5-6).

The hospital labor attorney and the industrial relations department should be prepared to take any necessary legal action. They should also explain the legal

Exhibit 5–3 Sample Victim Report

Date _____

Time _____

COMPANY CONFIDENTIAL

(To be completed in handwriting of victim of strike incident)

I, _____, of my own free will and without promise of reward, make the following statement regarding an incident that occurred during a strike by Local _____ during the month of _____.

I work in the _____; my foreman or supervisor is
                     (Location)

_____. I am ( ) am not ( ) (Check one) a member of Local _____.

The incident occurred at _____ A.M. ( ) P.M. ( ) (Check one) on the _____ day of _____ at the following location:
                          (Month and year)
_____.

The following persons whom I know witnessed the incident:
_____
_____

A brief description of the incident is as follows:
_____
_____
_____

I identify the following persons responsible for the incident:

Name	Department

As a result of the incident I suffered the following damage or injury: _____
Was medical treatment required? _____
If so, by whom? _____

Witness to signature

_____   _____
                                            Signature

situation to the strike management committee and the department heads at appropriate intervals. They should provide managers with the information they need to answer the questions of employees who have crossed the picket line to keep working.

When a pattern of violence occurs or entrance to the hospital is blocked consistently, the labor attorney should ask for police protection. The general duties of the police in strikes and labor disputes are the same as those under unusual

Exhibit 5–4 Sample Letter to Staff during Strike

Dear Staff Member:

As you are aware, the hospital and the union have been engaged in bargaining sessions since _____, in an attempt to arrive at a fair and equitable agreement satisfactory to both sides. Attached hereto is a summary of the final offer. Unfortunately, despite the efforts of both the union and the hospital, we are about to complete the _____ week in a strike situation without having reached an agreement. At our meeting yesterday, it became apparent that we have reached an impasse. There are no more meetings scheduled with the union negotiating committee, because they asked for our final offer and we gave them our final offer. There is no need to meet when there is an impasse.

The hospital, in order to protect its patients and give them the best care available, will start hiring permanent replacements for those on strike effective _____. Please regard this letter as an invitation to resume your regular position with the hospital on your regularly scheduled shift.

Wages and benefits, duties and obligations will be observed by both the hospital and those employees who return to work in accordance with the hospital's last offer to the union, which was voted upon and rejected by the union on _____.

If you fail to report on duty by _____, the hospital will be forced to seek a permanent replacement to fill your job. We hope you want to come back on duty, as we much prefer to operate with our present staff. A real issue will develop a few weeks from now when some of our present staff report for duty *after* they have been replaced by new employees. Now is the time to consider that.

We have been assured by the local law enforcement agencies and the union that there will be no violence on the picket line, so anyone who wants to return to work can do so.

We are hopeful that you will give proper consideration to this offer to return to your job. We are looking forward to seeing you and your fellow staff members back on duty so that you can give your patients the care to which they are entitled.

I urge you to contact your head nurse or our Personnel Manager, _____ _____ at the office or at their homes in regard to your plans so that we may arrange our health care scheduling.

Sincerely,

conditions of any type, i.e., to protect life and property and to maintain order. The existence of a labor problem does not license people to behave abnormally or to do things in groups that they cannot do individually. Sample general guidelines from the labor unit of a major city's police department are as follows:

- Picketing is legal if peacefully conducted.
- Picket lines shall form on sidewalks and shall confine themselves to the outside or curb side of the sidewalk so that anyone wishing to pass may do so freely.

Exhibit 5–5 Sample Press Release

The Good Hope Hospital submitted its final offer to the union on _____.
In wages and fringe benefits, the offer amounted to a _____% increase in the first year and a _____% increase in the second year.

The hospital administration was extremely disappointed that its final offer was not accepted, as it felt that the offer was fair and equitable for all concerned if the hospital is to remain competitive.

Negotiations have been broken off, and there are no further meetings scheduled.

- Pickets shall not form along streets or roads.
- A picket need not be a hospital employee.
- Unions may have as many pickets as they wish, provided that the pickets are peaceful and orderly.
- Pickets must keep moving.
- A picket line that stops or becomes unruly becomes a mob and is subject to arrest. A mob consists of five or more persons.
- People working in or having any business with a hospital in which employees are on strike have the right to pass freely; to enter or leave the hospital without being impeded, stopped, or threatened with bodily harm.
- Any person who wishes to take merchandise in or out of the hospital can do so without being impeded, stopped, or threatened with bodily harm.
- Pickets may not in any way block a door, passageway, driveway, crosswalk, or other entrance or exit to the struck hospital.
- Pickets may not impede traffic at the site of the strike.
- Union officials or pickets have the right to talk to people going in or out of the struck hospital, as long as they are orderly.
- A nonstriker who does not wish to talk to the union official or pickets is not required to do so and may go about freely without being stopped, impeded, intimidated, coerced, or threatened.
- Fighting, assault, battery, violence, threat, or intimidation is not permitted.
- Firearms, knives, clubs, and other weapons are not permitted.
- Pickets may stand alongside doors or entrances to pass out leaflets to persons entering and leaving the hospital, as long as they do not block the passageway.
- Sound trucks may be used if they are not too noisy and if the truck keeps moving.
- Profanity is not permitted.

Exhibit 5–6 Instructions to Employees in the Event of a Strike

1. All employees should report to work at their usual starting times.
2. Employees who drive to work should not drive alone during a strike. They should arrange to have at least one other employee in the car with them who could serve as a witness in the event of any incident occurring while crossing a picket line. Whenever possible, employees should form car pools for the duration of a strike. Among other things, this will simplify the traffic problem.
3. Employees entering plant property in automobiles should *roll their car windows up* and *lock their doors* before crossing picket lines.
4. In the event that pickets are parading or standing in front of cars, employees wishing to enter the plant should not try to force their way through the line, but should go slow and wait until there is an opening. If a Deputy Sheriff is stationed nearby, employees should ask assistance in driving through the line.
5. Employees entering on foot, if confronted by a tight picket line, should tell pickets that they are employees and that they wish to go to their jobs as is their legal right. If pickets should refuse to allow the employees to enter, the employees should seek the assistance of the local law enforcement authorities and, if possible, get the name or at least the descriptions of the pickets who denied them entrance. This information should be documented in detail and referred to Plant Protection.
6. An employee who is denied entrance or delayed in entering by illegal picketing should report this fact immediately to the supervisor who will arrange for the employee to make a sworn written statement covering the circumstances of the delay or denial. These statements, called affidavits, will be helpful to the hospital in gaining court injunction banning illegal picketing and should be referred to Plant Protection.
7. An employee who is injured or suffers injury to clothing or automobile while crossing the picket line should report this injury or damage immediately to the supervisor, who will arrange for the employee to make a statement of the damage or injury and take steps to gain reimbursement from the hospital for uninsured property damage.
8. If, in spite of all efforts, an employee is unable to cross a picket line to get to work, the employee should proceed to the nearest telephone and call the supervisor for further instructions. In these cases, the employee will probably be asked to make a statement, or affidavit, setting forth the circumstances that made it impossible for the employee to come to work. These statements can be used in securing a court injunction.
9. Employees may also take steps in their own behalf to protect their own individual rights:

   • An employee who is prevented from going to work by illegal mass picketing and suffers a pay loss as a result may wish to consult an attorney regarding the possibility of filing a lawsuit against the union for damages either individually or in company with other employees who suffered pay losses. The Supreme Court has held that the union may be held liable for such employee pay losses if the union prevents employees from coming to work by violence and threats of bodily harm on a picket line.

   • An employee who is physically assaulted by a picket while crossing the picket line has two courses of action open: (1) consult an attorney concerning the possibility of filing suit; and (2) swear out a complaint against the picket or pickets and have them arrested.

   • Employees who are subjected to offensive language, or to insulting, or threatening language or conduct may swear out a complaint against the individual or individuals responsible.

- A squad car may be necessary at the scene where there has been violence or serious threats.
- Picketing may be limited when there has been violence and subsequent legal action.

In addition to notifying the police of a strike, the employer should notify them of the:

- nature of the labor problem
- name of firm and others affected
- the location of the labor dispute
- the number of employees involved
- names and addresses of representatives of the union and the employer
- cause of the strike and any particular incidents
- whether police protection has been requested or granted.

The police should receive updates on the strike at least each week, unless there are incidents that warrant more frequent communication. The union, the police representative, the employer, and labor attorney should meet to discuss the plans and expectations of all parties.

Only if police protection is not given should a petition for an injunction be initiated. Under federal law (the Norris-LaGuardia Act) and many state acts, documentation of inadequate police protection is required before an injunction can be issued. Observers should be stationed at employee and patient entrances to document all acts of violence and mass picketing. Photographers should be recruited to take motion pictures and still shots *only* of unlawful conduct, such as mass picketing and violence. Taking pictures of peaceful picketing is unlawful (see *Puritana Mfg. Corp.,* 159 NLRB 518 [1966]).

All communications to the public, the union, and employees must be carefully monitored to ensure that they are devoid of statements that could be construed as unfair labor practices. Communications should emphasize factual information that builds morale of those supporting hospital operations during the strike. They should be short and factual, in keeping with the total strike plan, and reviewed by legal counsel.

CHECKLIST FOR HOSPITAL WHEN EMPLOYEES ARE TO STRIKE

Negotiations

1. Bargain offensively.
   - Go into negotiations totally prepared.

- Do not wait until union submits a proposal, start months ahead on the hospital's proposal, make reasonable requests, and back up positions with facts.
- Clarify strike issues.

2. Set reasonable goals for negotiations and back them up with facts.
3. Assume there will be a strike, and plan on what obstacles the hospital will encounter and how to overcome them.
4. Offer wages and fringe benefits in line with settlements in the industry and community.
5. Explain hospital positions to employees and supervisors. (Do supervisors feel they are part of management?)
6. Be brief, and factual, counter inaccuracies. If the hospital's positions are reasonable, stick to them.
7. Remember that the local union committee is made up of hospital employees; treat them as individuals.
8. Instruct employees in how to handle threatening calls and the picket lines.

Steps To Take during a Strike

1. Meet with police, prosecuting attorney, and union representative to establish ground rules for picket lines.
2. Establish complete *security plans;* hire an independent security force that specializes in security during labor disputes. Security is the single most important item in a strike for employees, patients, and the public.
   Consider the use of fence lighting, video tapes, parabolic microphones, Polaroid cameras (for all guards), and informants.
3. After first incident of mass picketing or violence, request a joint meeting with union, local committee, hospital representatives, and police to establish *ground rules* for picketing, e.g.:

   - Only two pickets at each entrance and exit.
   - Pickets continuously moving.
   - No verbal threats or name calling.
   - No weapons or other objects on picket line.

4. Keep a strike log.

   - All incidents must be logged as to date, time, place, person, or persons involved, and signed.
   - Use the military approach; namely, collect every bit of information possible and evaluate it to attempt to interpret the union's next move.

5. Make sure the supervisory staff is adequate to make up a mobile work strike force (key personnel) and is paid accordingly; if possible, make in-house arrangements for them so they do not have to cross the picket line.

6. Prepare ads for the public entitled "Your Right To Know," since public opinion wins long strikes.

7. Check telephones for listening devices.

8. Stockpile critical supplies.

9. Invest one central administrator with full authority and responsibility for support functions of the institution for the duration of the planning, strike, and poststrike periods. Disseminate all strike-related information rapidly through this central receiving point.

10. Set up a mobile force of one individual from each department (e.g., nursing, materials, dietary, purchasing, plant and facilities/maintenance, pharmacy, and housekeeping) to assist the person with authority to serve as strike coordinator.

11. Direct all communications between the planning group and the staff through the strike administrator.

12. Develop plans for security of supplies.

13. Alert all suppliers regarding possibility of a strike without providing details, and discuss alternative methods for continuation of service if they think their personnel would honor a picket line.

14. Have the director of purchasing develop a list of all major and key suppliers and see if they will cross picket lines with supervisor drivers, if necessary; identify what key pharmacy and dietary items must be kept on hand at all times; coordinate security for supply vehicles and storage areas with house security.

15. Obtain assistance from outside sources, such as other hospitals, suppliers, and service agents, if possible.

16. Consider an outside warehouse facility to serve as a drop point for deliveries. It is a must to review and discuss with suppliers the need for drop shipments *before* they are placed so that pickets turning away sympathetic drivers will be kept to a minimum.

17. Build up inventory only of absolutely essential items.

18. Because it will be demoralizing to strikers to see suppliers' vehicles and other service trucks continuing routine deliveries to hospital, provide for a pool of trucks and vans, either owned or leased by the hospital, and employees to drive them to augment suppliers' deliveries.

19. Determine the census needed to maintain an economic balance to pay the salaries of hospital personnel during a strike.

20. Establish a strike communications center and command post.

21. Explain the official position of the hospital to supervisory personnel and security forces, as well as what they can and cannot say concerning the status of negotiations. Ask their opinions.

22. Discharge as many patients as possible.
23. Consolidate remaining patients.
24. Decide whether to keep the emergency room open.
25. Provide extra security and police the first few days of strike, when strikers are greatest in number and most exuberant.
26. Establish ground rules from Day one. Do not compromise—employees still must obey the law.
27. Be ready for union propaganda that it is dangerous to be a patient in a struck hospital.

NOTES

1. Bureau of National Affairs, "Selected Materials Distributed at Conference on Organizing Women Workers," *Daily Labor Report,* 29 January 1981.

2. Bonnie Castrey and Robert Castrey, "Mediation—What It Is, What It Does," *Journal of Nursing Administration* 10 (November 1980): 24–28.

3. Stephen Cabot and Jerald Cureton, "Labor Disputes and Strikes: Be Prepared," *Personnel Journal* 60 (February 1981): 121–123, 136.

4. Castrey and Castrey, "Mediation."

5. Robert Coulson, *Labor Arbitration: What You Need to Know* (New York: American Arbitration Association, 1978).

6. Franklin Schaffer, "A 70-Day Strike by Professional Nurses," *Supervisor Nurse* 11 (September 1980): 49–54.

Chapter 6

Grievances and Arbitration

Since the passage of Public Law 93–360 (Health Care Amendments of 1974), resulting in more active involvement of hospitals in labor relations, many hospitals have written improved policies and rules. These documents usually include statements on employee conduct and duties, as well as on wages, benefits, and other conditions of employment. Administrators are learning that these documents and their implementation, or lack of implementation, become the track record of so-called past practice on which court decisions are based.

Hospitals are ripe for grievances because of their labor-intensive nature. Sparks of conflict are even more likely because women and minorities are overrepresented in the hospital work force. Decentralization further complicates matters, as middle managers are only beginning to have adequate skills and theory to implement an equitable, enlightened policy of employee relations. In addition, managers are continually faced with the thorny communication problems fostered by the highly interdependent nature of professional groups and departments in a hospital.

While grievance procedures have traditionally been confined to unionized settings, some union-free hospitals have begun to formalize their complaint-handling methods. A Communigram complaint program (see in Chapter 8) is for a union-free setting—one of the more important features being that the physicians' group is involved in the complaint process in an attempt to make physicians responsible for their acts, which is an area of real concern for a number of different groups in a hospital. Some union-free hospitals even include a hearing by an impartial review board in the complaint procedure so that employees may be assured of equitable treatment.

CONTRACT ADMINISTRATION

In those hospitals where employees are unionized and a contract has been signed, employees are typically able to use a well-delineated grievance procedure that includes arbitration.

Cooperative Approach

For many hospital administrators and nurse-managers, contract administration in a unionized hospital is a new experience. Successful contract administration requires a management team with a contingency approach, one that is flexible according to situational demands and allows managers to be responsive to staff input in the form of needs, concerns, complaints, and suggestions for change. So as not to lose meaningful direction, the management team needs a pragmatic philosophy and a realistic grasp of departmental objectives as they relate to all employees. Top level managers need to equip front line managers with the knowledge and skills necessary to implement a contemporary management philosophy. Finally, managers must encourage participatory decision making and recognition for staff members who expend extra effort to benefit co-workers or to improve patient care.

THE UNION REPRESENTATIVE

As the majority representative of the employees in a bargaining unit, the union representative must be consulted when scheduled hours, shifts, holidays, vacations, leaves, or weekends are to be changed unless the hospital has specifically retained its management rights to unilaterally make such changes in the collective bargaining agreement. Other changes in wages, hours, and working conditions that affect employees must also be discussed with the union representative. Early involvement of the union representative in the change is a good step in cushioning employee response to change and in avoiding grievances. The important point to distinguish is that the union representative is called in only *after* the management decision is made and is not allowed in the actual decision-making process.

While a cordial working relationship with the union is desirable, managers must remember that the union exists because employees were dissatisfied with their ability to communicate with management. The employees pay the union to represent them. To remain in existence, the union must convince employees that the union gets concessions that employees could not get by themselves. Thus, managers should not be surprised when rumors of a successful union-management meeting are favorable to the union. Such slanted reporting may anger and frustrate managers. Top management must maintain a close supportive relationship with the front line managers, who now have an extra layer of bureaucracy with which to cope.

The union representative who sides too often with management will become distrusted by employees. Thus, some conflict in union-management relations is unavoidable. When the union representative is reasonable and competent, management should try to avoid the ouster of that representative; the next one might be more militant and difficult.

Committees

Many labor contracts make provisions for committees on practice in which the union is also represented. Committees such as the nursing practice or joint practice committees can be a forum in which managers can take the pulse of the hospital, provided that committee meetings do not become just grievance meetings. Input obtained from these meetings can be used in decision making that improves employee working conditions and patient care. Typically, nursing practice committees deal with issues such as safety, quality assurance, patient care standards, and patient classification systems. Joint practice committees usually tackle the thorny problems of nurse-physician relations.

COMMON ISSUES IN A FIRST CONTRACT

The most common problem areas in a first contract are supervisors working, job ownership, recognition of the union, job bidding, and overtime.

Supervisors Working

In non-health care settings, it is not unusual for a conflict over supervisors working to cause a wildcat strike.

As hospitals are different from most businesses, the supervisor is as much a clinical consultant as an administrator. Because this role takes both nursing and management skills, it is very stressful and requires a great deal of contact with patient care. Management skills may be increased at the expense of clinical skills in the rapidly changing acute care setting. Still, on weekends and second and third shifts, supervisors are called upon to do much of what they have done for years. Even during the day shift, supervisors may be required to lend a hand, since it is not always possible to predict some of the crises that can occur in hospitals. For this reason, it is imperative that hospitals insist on a clause in the contract that allows supervisors to continue with the past practices of their positions.

Supervisors delve into the work of the bargaining unit most often when a care provider, patient, or visitor has a behavioral outburst, when an emergency occurs; when mealtime or break time replacements are unavailable; or when no bargaining unit member is available to replace an absent employee. They also involve themselves in providing direct patient care to keep their skills current, to solve a patient care problem, or to set an example for staff members who are being informally or formally apprenticed. Such hands-on competence has always been encouraged in the profession of nursing, since it is a way of passing on skills from the experienced professionals to less skilled practitioners. Hospitals must not agree to a union clause against supervisors working in any health care setting as, among other things, it would discourage hospitals from hiring expert practitioners to improve the practice and delivery of health care services.

Job Ownership

Under a union contract when an employee is asked to "float" to another area or to assist another team member in finishing an assignment, sparks often fly with the employee saying, "that's not my job." As long as seniority clauses are only the basis for general promotions, employees may not refuse to move to another job, provided that doing so is not a violation of licensing laws or practice acts within the state. Seniority does not give an employee the right to pick a job or refuse to float unless you agree to this in a collective bargaining agreement. The hospital can be better protected in such a situation by having the following contract language:

> The hospital in its discretion may assign any employee to perform duties that normally fall in any other job classification, as long as state laws or licensing regulations are not violated, in order to meet operating require-ments, or to make efficient use of an employee's services.

Unions typically fight this type of provision in a contract. To operate efficiently, however, hospitals have always had to make staff assignments in accordance with their needs. Because more lawsuits are involving nurses who have been sent to areas in which they are not oriented and competent to work, many hospitals are training their nurses to work in several like areas.[1] Thus, when the patient census falls on one unit and rises in another, the hospital can float help to the area of need. Management should fight union attempts to control this process.

Job ownership also creates problems when job descriptions are used. Never include job descriptions in any collective bargaining agreement. However, if you do provide job descriptions, they should be written in terms of "levels of work expectations" as an aid in performance appraisals, not an ironclad sign of job ownership. The last statement of a job description must be purposefully open-ended to avoid such rigidity in employee interpretation.

There has been a great deal of discussion on job ownership as unions and state nurses' associations constantly raise such issues as the use of outside agency nurses to fill staffing gaps and the assignment of staff nurses to higher rated jobs for a few days. For example, if both the head nurse and the assistant are gone from the hospital and the contract does not stipulate a charge rate premium for as little as one shift, a staff nurse is generally allowed to assume the position for as short a period as possible. Otherwise, it might be necessary to pay the staff nurse a salary that belongs to a different classification.

Problems in calculating responsibility will increase as more health care institu-tions move from centralized to decentralized operations. In some totally decentralized settings, everyone and no one can be in charge because the coordinator spot rotates. In many settings, however, it is not uncommon to see one unit making total patient care assignments while others switch between team nursing and total patient care in accord with the personalities involved. There is often no reason for discrepancies in the method, since the concept of assignments is in transition to the point that nurses vary in their understanding both of assignment methods and of the meaning of being in charge. Thus, hospitals should not agree to narrow job definitions or any other clause in the labor agreement that interferes with the rotation of nurses or with the team nursing concept.

Recognition of the Union

The feelings of managers and staff members about the events and emotions that were part of the union organizing effort must be put aside. The hospital's goal must be to work on peaceful coexistence with the union. The union represents the employees. Management's objective is to retain all of its rights without being combative. As the employer, the hospital must train all supervisors in labor relations, implement a sound program designed to maintain the dignity of the individual employee, and meet the needs of employees while providing the best patient care possible.

Every manager should know the terms of the contract and should work to base all decisions on facts and positions supportable under the law in order to minimize the number of grievances. Arbitration is a time-consuming, costly process that can also have a negative effect on public relations, depending on the issues, the outcomes, and their subsequent coverage by the media.[2]

Job Bidding

A union often makes some provision for nurses in the bargaining unit to get preferred shifts or promotions on the basis of their seniority. It may be unwise to give shift preferences on the basis of seniority. However, in promotion management must always make the initial determination of whether an individual has the skill and ability to do the job. If a job is not to be given to a nurse in the bargaining unit who should get it by seniority, management should interview the employee and document the reasons that management feels the employee cannot handle the position. If the reasons for not giving the job to that employee are marginal, managers may wish to allow that employee a trial period (not a training period) on the job or shift to prove that he or she is capable of doing the job.

Overtime

A big bone of contention in hospitals is overtime. Mandatory overtime is an inherent management right that must not be surrendered. Many contracts are quite specific on the conditions of overtime and may include some type of statement requiring that overtime be offered to regular employees before agency nurses are utilized. As time and one-half is given for overtime, hospital managers run into problems. If the contract is not carefully worded, staff members drawing on-call pay or overtime money can make more than the managers, a situation demoralizing to managers.

In one hospital, it was agreed that nurses would receive double pay for working one complete second shift in a twenty-four hour period. Because the nursing shortage in this hospital was critical and per diem nurses held out until they were promised a double shift, the per diem nurses were able to make more money doing two double shifts per week than the full-time nurses who were also required to work weekends and holidays. This overtime problem caused low morale for full-time employees, uncomfortable working relationships for per diem people, and undue blame on management.

GRIEVANCES

It is important for managers to understand the difference between a grievance and a complaint. A grievance is usually interpreted as a violation of contract provisions, while a complaint refers to any other type of conflict. A complaint may become a grievance if the application or interpretation of the contract is the cause of the problem or if the employee takes issue with arbitrary, capricious, or discriminatory decision making by a supervisor. A grievance procedure is a quasi-judicial procedure for resolving disputes and misunderstandings.

Prevention of Grievances

Probably the single most important way to avoid grievances is for managers to get to know the employees and to take a sincere interest in them. Supervisors should be sure to speak to employees daily, calling them by name and showing a genuine concern for their aspirations, problems, needs and concerns as individuals. It is necessary to show a sense of humor with them as well. In mingling with employees, supervisors should be receptive to their ideas and comments, and should follow up on them in such a way that they know their input matters. While trying to be friendly with employees, managers should guard against intimacy with employees, which can create problems with the working relationship. The employee who has worked extra hard should be given credit. People need to be acknowledged for what they do; too often, employees become discouraged because what they are doing does not seem to matter to anyone.

Good managers spend the lion's share of their time in listening. By listening intently and empathetically to employees, a manager often finds that the employee either talks the problem out or continues to talk until the *real* problem surfaces. Then the manager can work toward an effective solution. Whenever an employee confides in a manager, it is critical for the manager to respect that confidence. Employees watch managers very carefully to see if a trusting relationship is possible.

In listening to employees, it is important to be open-minded. Sometimes the problem that the employee is experiencing can be corrected through better in-service training or through modification of a form or a procedure. The employee does not always understand why things are not going along as smoothly as they should. The manager can help by bringing the resources of the hospital to the aid of the employee, once the problem-solving method has been applied to the situation.

The supervisor who works to avoid grievances can be most effective by working to resolve the problem quickly so that small problems do not snowball into large ones:

1. Determine the cause of the employee's dissatisfaction.
2. Seek to understand the employee's perception of the situation.
3. Discuss the problem objectively with the employee.
4. Obtain data from other people, managers, and past practices of the hospital to clarify the problem and the possible solutions.
5. Evaluate the solutions in light of the contract, possible precedents, cost, and effect on others.
6. Implement a solution that minimizes the irritation. If a solution is not known or a change in policy is not feasible, be sure to inform the employee at least about the follow-up and the rationale for the final decision.

Many grievances arise from "the people things." It is not *what* employees must do in the work setting, but *how* they are asked to do it. Often, the attitude of others makes a job difficult and unpleasant. For example, in one situation, an extremely popular staff nurse who was given a supervisory position developed such an air of self-importance when she assumed the job that the morale of the employees deteriorated. It is fair to say that most supervisors go through a phase of feeling important, but successful supervisors soon develop the proper sense of perspective.

Favoritism is a major cause of grievances. Like anyone else, managers like certain people and dislike others. In spite of their personal feelings, managers must remain sensitive to the needs of all employees and work hard to be fair. When managers are not equitable in their dealings with employees, everyone soon knows it. Hard feelings over unequal treatment surface in any number of undesirable ways.

In talking with the union representative about a problem, managers should listen attentively without taking personal offense at what they are hearing. The problem-solving method can be used to advantage. The union representative will talk to involved employees, and the manager should plan to talk with them, too, so that they can see the manager's concern for their needs. Such a conversation must be evaluated in relation to the specific situation and to the whole picture. Often, the initial complaint is merely the tip of the iceberg.

The Supervisor As a Source of Grievances

When a hospital is newly unionized, supervisors often resent having their decisions questioned and being required to answer to the union. They may take one of two approaches in their management style. In the first, they may become "bossy," ordering employees to obey directions; without giving any reasons for such orders but with an attitude of "you'll do it because I'm the boss." Of course, highly skilled and professional employees resent this method. In the second extreme approach, they may become weak, allowing employees to "get away" with things, causing employees to lose respect for them, and setting a very bad precedent for other supervisors. There are several points that supervisors should consider as they work to minimize grievances.

Anger. When a supervisor administers discipline during a moment of temper, the decision and methods selected are often less appropriate than usual and indefensible by objective standards.

Promises. As an agent of management, supervisors should not make any promises that they cannot keep and are not willing to fulfill for all employees. Promises should seldom be made to employees; if promises are made, however, they should be kept. Otherwise, the employees will feel that they have grounds for a grievance. Supervisors should be careful not to make any statements that could be interpreted as a promise.

Additional suggestions for effective labor relations for preventive maintenance of complaints and arbitrations can be found in Appendix 6-A.

Types of Employees

One of the most difficult problems for a supervisor is to determine the best way to deal with each employee. Each has a different personality, and an approach that is effective in dealing with one will not work at all in dealing with another. For instance, Tom may be the outgoing, excitable type who makes his position clear immediately; if upset, he states his problem, usually calms down quickly, and discusses the problem in a rational manner. In contrast, Mary may be a quiet, introspective, serious type who seems always to have control of her emotions and seldom shows any outward evidence that she is displeased. If Mary explodes, however, it will take time to solve her problem. Of these two extreme types, managers find it easier to deal with Tom, because they are aware immediately that

Tom has a gripe. The problem elicited from Mary, however, will have to be drawn out by the manager. The supervisor must treat Tom calmly so as not to aggravate the emotional climate. For Mary, on the other hand, the supervisor will probably have to wait quite a while before she will reveal her problem, and the supervisor will have to be sensitive in helping her. These are two extremes. Most employees are a combination of Tom and Mary. It is clear, however, that supervisors must evaluate the personalities and temperaments of their subordinates in order to determine the most effective way to deal with each one. For example, a supervisor should know when and how to use praise to obtain the desired result in dealing with a certain employee and whether a certain employee will respond more readily to a challenge or to objective criticism. There is no substitute for knowing employees as individuals.

Discipline

Another major area that breeds grievances is discipline. When a contract is in effect, it is improper to take a contractual benefit away from an employee as a part of discipline. Furthermore, management should not refuse to promote an employee because of absenteeism, even if the contract cites dependability as a factor in determining qualifications. An arbitrator might find *double jeopardy* in such a situation. In other words, not only are employees disciplined for their absenteeism, but also this absenteeism record is used to withhold a promotion. Arbitrators have ruled both ways in various cases where double jeopardy is an issue.

It is also very important to avoid terminating an employee immediately. If the disciplinary policy requires progressive discipline, supervisors should adhere to it. If the rule violation is one that warrants immediate dismissal, the employee should be suspended until a complete investigation has been done. Such an investigation provides the supervisor with time to regain emotional composure and to process the case in a way that best protects management's position. At times, the employee is shown to be not guilty of the infraction first suspected, and the final outcome can be quite different from the outcome had action been taken at once.

Arbitrators do not generally treat insubordination as a dischargeable offense unless it is a direct refusal of a clearly defined order and there is no problem with safety. Management must define the discipline appropriate for different types of behavior. When an employee has a generally poor record of performance, it is sometimes better to concentrate on the most serious problem in the corrective interviews and in the documentation in that area. Otherwise, it may appear to an arbitrator that management has discriminated against the employee by using weak trivial incidents.

The supervisor must know what to do when an employee requests a union steward. It was held in *NLRB v. Weingarten, Inc.*, 420 U.S. 251 (1974) that employees have the right to have a union steward present when interviews are "investigatory" and "disciplinary," but not when the sole purpose of a meeting is to notify an employee of previously decided discipline. Objective standards rather than an employee's subjective motivations are used to determine whether an employee *reasonably* believes the interview might result in disciplinary action. Under Weingarten, the employee must request union representation. However, if an employee is simply refusing an assignment, he or she is not entitled to union representation and the "work now, grieve later" principle applies; thus the employee must do the assigned work unless a safety issue is involved, as ruled in *Whirlpool Corp. v. Marshall,* 100 S.Ct. 883 (1980). If the employee continues to refuse the assignment, the supervisor should ask for the employee's union steward and another management representative to witness a repeated request and refusal. Even in this case, however, the employer does not need to notify the union steward if the employee has not requested the steward's presence.

The following three situations provide some guidelines for disciplining employees.

1. If the manager is merely giving an oral warning and the employee asks for the union steward, the manager should *stop the interview and go no further.*
2. If an employee is to be given more than an oral warning for refusing to do a job and the manager is going to ask questions about the employee's refusal to do the job, the manager should bring a management witness and a union steward, if one is requested by the employee.
3. If the manager is only going to give notice of disciplinary action already decided and is not going to ask any questions or discuss any matters, the manager need not grant the request for a union steward.

Anytime a manager feels that an employee is likely to bring a discrimination suit, the manager should bring in another supervisor to witness the conversation. When a union is on the scene, it is doubly important to follow the hospital disciplinary policy rigidly and to check with labor relations or personnel on rules and policies so that enforcement can be consistent for all employees. Furthermore, managers must document all discipline administered and the reasons for it at the time the incident happens. This documentation, as well as that for all statements made by the employee, should be placed in the employee record.

If an employee wants to see his or her personnel record, the manager should:

- ask the employee what information is needed, and answer any questions that the employee has
- allow the employee to view a specific item in the record (if doing so is a simple request), but not to peruse the entire file freely
- seek advice from the hospital's labor attorney in important or sensitive cases

If necessary, the manager should tell the employee that the record is the property of the hospital. In almost no case should the manager turn over the personnel file to the employee. This is based on the fact that the employee's personnel file is the exclusive property of the hospital that compiled it, and the employee has no property rights to his or her file either to look at it or to demand copies of documents in it even though the documents in the file relate to the employee.

At present only the following states, California, Maine, Michigan, Oregon, Pennsylvania, Connecticut, and Wisconsin have enacted laws permitting employee access to personnel files. For example, laws in Pennsylvania and Maine allow employees to review their personnel files at reasonable times during normal office hours. In Wisconsin, employees must be permitted to view their files within seven days of a request. Employees in Connecticut and Michigan can challenge information in the file, limit the information an employer may release, and require the employer to provide copies of specific items in the file. Managers in all states are advised to keep their records in good order, since this trend of allowing access to personnel files appears to be extending to the federal government and other states.

Handling Grievances

When a formal, written grievance is received, the supervisor should:

1. Date and initial the grievance, showing exactly when it was received. Under a typical labor agreement, the employee must present a grievance within a stipulated number of working days of the employee's knowledge of it. If the grievance is untimely, the supervisor should accept it, but write "Not valid grievance—untimely."
2. Make sure the employee has signed the grievance.
3. Ensure that the grievance includes the paragraphs of the agreement alleged to have been violated, if required.
4. Ensure that the grievance contains a statement of the facts that have given rise to the alleged grievance.
5. Determine what the union is asking for by way of remedy.
6. Refuse to extend time limits unless for a very good cause. Failure to adhere to time limits establishes a very bad precedent.
7. Make an investigation and talk to any witnesses, making notes of the investigation to give to the personnel department. Notes should be precise to the point of exact quotes.
8. Put "No contract violation" if unsure how to answer the grievance.
9. Be consistent with other departments in the grievance.

Cases of Discharge

An employee who is being suspended for a rule that does not automatically require termination in appropriate cases should be told that the hospital will reinstate him or her on certain conditions. Under these conditions, the suspension will be treated as a disciplinary layoff if the hospital, union, and employee sign a letter of understanding. Such a final letter or memorandum of understanding should include the following points:

1. a brief statement of the reason for the employee's suspension
2. a statement that the agreement to reinstate the employee cannot be used as a precedent for disciplinary violations by other employees
3. an acknowledgement that the hospital has been lenient in this incident and the disciplinary action taken was warranted and justified
4. an admission that the employee understands his or her past overall performance as an employee with the hospital has been "unacceptable" and recognizes the second opportunity to correct this condition
5. a statement that the employee realizes that disregarding this memorandum of understanding or commiting serious violation of other hospital rules will result in termination of employment
6. a statement that the employee has read the above and understands it completely

The document should be dated and signed, with titles, by the supervisor and the employee involved, a member from personnel, and the union representative(s) who participated in the reinstatement conference.

ARBITRATION

Some union-free hospitals have an ombudsperson who works as an independent agent in resolving conflicts and complaints. These hospitals may provide employees with the opportunity to submit grievances under the Expedited Employment Arbitration Rules of the American Arbitration Association.[3] This system is activated when the employee has exhausted the usual steps of a complaint procedure, i.e., discussing the grievance with the supervisor, receiving an oral answer, presenting the grievance to the supervisor in writing, and continuing with the written grievance if the problem has not been resolved. At this stage the personnel department and the administration receive the grievance and determine the final position of the hospital. This position is put into writing. The grievant may continue by requesting an arbitration hearing held before an impartial arbitrator appointed by the American Arbitration Association under its Expedited Rules. No briefs are filed, and no recorded transcripts are kept. The arbitrator renders a decision within five working days, which may be posted on the bulletin board. In 1976, the American Arbitration Association published a casebook of arbitration awards involving the health care industry that provides insight into the types of issues that have been arbitrated and the ensuing decisions.[4]

When a hospital is unionized, the grievance arbitration procedure is usually specified in the contract. When there are problems in understanding, applying, or interpreting the contract, the union typically takes precedential cases to arbitration. Discharges are also taken to arbitration usually. The introduction of formal arbitration into the health care field has caused many managers to realize the need for more sophistication in the handling of employees. Most experts feel that the number of arbitration cases in health care will increase because of the contemporary pressures of inflation, cost containment, and the need for increased productivity. Precedents established during arbitration not only affect the hospital involved, but also have industrywide effects.

The American Arbitration Association is a public service, membership corporation that was established in 1926 as a means of encouraging arbitration and like techniques as a voluntary means to settle disputes. Most union contracts contain a clause that allows grievances to end in binding arbitration as a quid pro quo for the union's no-strike pledge.

Each grievance is a unique situation that varies according to the specific contract language, the relationship of the involved parties, and past practices of both parties. Some grievances are insignificant; others involve issues important for either the union or the hospital. The grievance procedure varies from contract to contract but the contract should be carefully worded so that the procedure meets the needs of the hospital and the union. The union takes as many cases to arbitration as it can afford, or for political reasons such as placating a particularly militant union steward. Most others are settled at a lower step of the grievance procedure.

The decisions of arbitrators are binding and may include an award of back pay or reinstatement of a discharged employee. Sometimes the award sets a precedent that will cost the hospital a great deal of money in the future. Because arbitrators sometimes exhibit personal biases, it is critical to investigate the arbitrator's background before a final selection is made. The hospital's labor attorney should have an arbitrator's biography that gives all the arbitrator's past decisions, shows whether the arbitrator exhibited any bias and whether the decisions were justified by the facts, includes the arbitrator's work history to show expertise in labor relations, and lists the professional associations to which the arbitrator belongs, such as the National Academy of Arbitrators (NAA).

Hospitals should settle for nothing less than an arbitrator who is in the NAA; if possible, this criterion should be written into the labor agreement.[5]

Those arbitrators who have been admitted to the NAA are experienced arbitrators who have made fifty or more decisions and have such a high professional reputation that they have been recommended for admission by both management and unions.

Managers who are preparing a case for arbitration should take the following steps:

1. Review the grievance procedure to date.
   - Read carefully all steps.
   - Review any minutes of meetings in the various steps.
   - Tell counsel all the union claims or defenses raised in grievance procedure.
   - Confirm that the grievance is timely and arbitrable.
2. Determine what the contract says on the issue involved.
3. Review correspondence in submitting dispute to arbitration.
4. Consider possible witnesses, both for the hospital and for the union, and their testimony.
   - Who made the final decision on the disciplinary action taken?
   - On what was the decision based?
   - Who actually witnessed facts essential to prove the case?
5. Interview all witnesses.
   - Go over with them their demeanor at the hearing.
   - Find out facts (what union is claiming, as well as what the hospital is claiming).
   - Prepare them for possible cross-examination.
6. Prepare list of exhibits and who will sponsor each exhibit.
7. Examine location where incident took place, if that is in any way relevant; determine if the arbitrator should view the site.
8. Consider the use of statistical or pictorial exhibits.
9. Compare past practice in similar situations, e.g., whether lesser discipline was administered for the same violation in the past.
10. Determine if the case will turn on a key point; if so, concentrate on that point.
11. Research prior arbitration cases on point involved to see what other arbitrators have considered on similar issues.
12. Prepare outline of case.
    - Opening statement
    - Order of witnesses
    - Order of presentation of exhibits (if possible)
      1. contract

   2. hospital rules
   3. grievance
13. Prepare expected questions and answers for witnesses to examine, but not to memorize.
14. Determine if any employees should be subpoenaed to avoid union retaliation for voluntary testimony.
15. If disciplinary case, review and make copies of all prior disciplinary actions taken against employee and any grievances filed over past disciplinary actions.
16. Review employee personnel file.
17. Consider whether some facts should be stipulated or whether live testimony is preferable.
18. If the case is complex, prepare a prehearing brief.
19. Determine whether the grievant or union made any admissions, either at the time of the incident or thereafter, that indicate guilt.
20. Prepare a brief description of the hospital's background, e.g., the number of employees in the bargaining unit and the history of the collective bargaining relationship.
21. Review files and arbitration awards involving the same parties that would have bearing on present case, as well as files and awards of similar cases.
22. Consider whether negotiations history has a bearing on the case, i.e., is the union trying to gain through arbitration what it was unable to obtain at the bargaining table?
23. Prepare for cross-examination of union's witnesses.
24. Frame the issue.
25. Arrange for a court reporter so that a transcript of everything that is said at the arbitration hearing will be available. Usually if it is an important enough issue to take to arbitration it is important enough to have a certified transcript, particularly if you have to challenge the Arbitrator's Award in federal district court.*

Are You a Credible Witness?

Being a good witness is paramount in winning any legal case for the hospital. Many health care managers are very anxious when they must testify in court or at an arbitration hearing. A witness takes an oath to tell the truth, however, if a

---

*The film—*The Supervisor and Arbitration* (Bureau of Business Practices, 24 Rope Ferry Road, Waterford, Connecticut 06386)—shows actual arbitration cases over documented grievances pointing out the five leading reasons why disciplinary penalties are very often reversed at arbitration. Your supervisors see key ingredients that are missing. As a result, your supervisors are able to plug these lax areas to build their penalties on a more solid foundation (16mm. film; color; modern).

witness falters and stumbles, an arbitrator, judge, or jury may wonder if the witness is indeed telling the truth. Thus, a witness must be confident and straightforward in giving testimony. Witnesses may find the following tips helpful:

1. Make your attorney go over the actual questions that are going to be asked at the hearing. Preferably, the questions should be written out before it is necessary to testify and they should be thoroughly reviewed well in advance of the hearing.
2. Before testifying, return to the site of the incident and review the details including a review of all distances between persons or equipment involved in the incident.
3. Dress in conservative clothes for the court appearance.
4. Avoid chewing gum or exhibiting nervous habits.
5. Be bold when taking the oath, and pay close attention to the proceedings.
6. Avoid memorizing testimony.
7. Remain serious at all times.
8. Avoid talking about the case in the halls or restrooms.
9. When answering questions in a jury trial, look directly at the jury. In arbitration, look at the arbitrator.
10. Speak to the jury and arbitrator as if they were friends.
11. Do not cover face or mouth when speaking.
12. Speak in a loud, clear voice so that the arbitrator, judge, or jury can easily hear and understand.
13. Be certain that you understand the question, if you don't, make them repeat the question; do not be distracted if the attorney for the other side is extremely friendly or rude.
14. After the question is repeated, take the time to give a considered, thoughtful answer.
15. Avoid pausing so long with each question that you appear to be making up answers.
16. Explain the answers as succinctly as possible. If the question on cross-examination is not a simple "yes" or "no" type, don't offer anything but fact, as your attorney on redirect will ask you the right questions.
17. Be certain to answer only the question being asked; do not volunteer information. For example, *Question:* Why did you discriminate against the employee? *Answer:* I didn't but we had an argument on the first day he came under my supervision.
18. Correct any wrong answer as quickly as possible.
19. If the answer is not understood, be sure to clarify it.
20. Don't editorialize. For example, "I know why you are asking me that question." Do not make statements about conclusions, opinions, or secondhand information; give only the facts.

21. End important accounts of the facts with a statement "That is all that I recall at this time," leaving the door open for more information at a later point.
22. No matter what feelings remain about prior events, the behavior of other parties, or the manner of the other attorney, be courteous.
23. Do not act cocky or obnoxious.
24. Do not try to decide when testifying if the truth will hurt or help the case, just give the facts. If the case has been prepared correctly, you won't be confronted with such a situation.
25. Avoid exaggerations.
26. If you do not know an answer, say so.
27. Avoid becoming emotional, as emotional witnesses may make remarks on cross-examination that will greatly hurt their credibility.
28. Trust the hospital's attorney to know when to object to a question, do not make this decision personally, do not ask advice of the judge.
29. Avoid hedging or arguing with the other attorney.
30. Discuss intricate details of conversations, hospital procedures, or other matters with the attorney prior to testifying so that your memory of the events is reasonable.
31. If the opposing attorney asks with whom you have discussed the case, if you have discussed the case with your attorney state that you have, and when you are asked what the attorney told you to say; testify that you were told to tell the truth and that by telling the truth there wasn't any way the case could be lost.

In summary, witnesses should be the type of honest, forthright person that they would believe if they were the arbitrator, judge, or jury.

NOTES

1. Helen Creighton, "Liability of Nurse Floated to Another Unit," *Nursing Management* 13(March 1982):54.

2. Robert Coulson, *Labor Arbitration—What You Need to Know,* 2d ed. (New York: American Arbitration Society, 1978).

3. Ibid.

4. American Arbitration Association, *Labor Arbitration in Health Care* (New York: American Arbitration Association, 1976).

5. Ibid.

Appendix 6-A

Effective Labor Relations for Preventive Maintenance of Complaints and Arbitrations

Chances are that, if you have already implemented some of the techniques discussed in this book and are actively considering more ways to do so, you have a great start on promoting a strong, positive image to your employees. In review, consider your position on the following points:

1. Do you avoid management by surprises? In other words, do employees "get the word" in an understandable way when you are making major changes or promoting major programs that affect (a) how you operate, (b) relationships between management and employees, or (c) the general status of the organization?
2. Are you tuned in to the needs of your employees for recognition and self-esteem?
3. What do you do to keep morale high?
4. Is your disciplinary policy fair and uniformly applied?
5. Do employees have a clear understanding of what you expect in terms of appropriate behaviors and adequate job performance?
6. Do you discharge employees that do unsatisfactory work or continually drag others down with a chronic negative attitude?
7. How credible are your efforts to promote employee rights?
8. Do you have an open door policy and a complaint system that *really* works?
9. How effective is your communication network in promoting upward, downward, and lateral communication?
10. Do employees know how you utilize their ideas in the management process and in future programs and policies for the organization?

Source: Arthur D. Rutkowski, *Working Together* (Evansville, Ind.: Aztec Printers, 1981); Barbara Lang Rutkowski, *Nursing Leadership: Challenges and Dilemmas* (Evansville, Ind.: Nurse Consultation Services, 1982).

11. Are you competitive in wages and fringe benefits?
12. Do you stay informed about employee policies and programs offered by your competitors?
13. How workable is your career ladder?
14. What training/education do you provide to upgrade employee skills to allow reimbursement of tuition costs for their continuing education credits (CEUs)?
15. What wage/benefits/incentives do you have for the nurse who deserves promotion but does not want to be a manager?
16. How do you rate on

- allowing nurses to be on joint practice and patient care committees?*
- creative and equitable staffing patterns?
- incentives to staff difficult periods, such as holidays, weekends, or night shift?
- granting leaves of absence that do not interrupt seniority?
- defining policies for seniority and promotion?
- providing continuing education and tuition reimbursement plans?
- providing accessible child care services?
- utilizing peer review?
- establishing guidelines/qualifications that govern staffing policies and patterns, especially in circumstances that require "float" nurses?

NOTES

---

*Joyce Riffer, "Pilot Program in Maine Hospital Shows How Nurses, Physicians Can Collaborate," *Hospitals* 55(November 1981): 17-24.

Chapter 7

Decertification

Hospitals, faced with lowered productivity and employees disenchanted with union representation, are in a good position in the 1980s to decertify their unions. The first step in the process of decertification is to learn what can and cannot be done.

MAKING THE DECISION

Is decertification worth the time, effort, and money? Hospitals which the union has caused few problems may decide that the presence of the union is not obtrusive enough to warrant the cost of decertification. Others, realizing that their management is not responsive to the needs of workers and does not practice effective labor relations, may feel that decertification of one union would leave employees open to another, even less desirable union. Each hospital must carefully analyze its own situation to determine the advantages and disadvantages of its current union-management relationship.

Managers should approach the idea of decertifying a union as rationally as they would any other business decision. Prior to beginning the decertification process, managers need to

1. make a commitment to the personal and organizational effort and costs required
2. be prepared to work tirelessly to establish effective working relationships with employees
3. negotiate and compromise with employees to prevent negative attitudes after the decertification process is over,
4. be prepared to face untoward outcomes related to the failure of an attempt at decertification[1,2,3]

THE PROCEDURE

There are three main procedures for deunionization: (1) the decertification petition (RD), (2) the deauthorization petition (UD), and (3) the employer petition (RM). The acronyms for these processes have been derived from NLRB casehandling procedures over the years and are commonly used in the labor relations literature.

Decertification Petition

When employees approach management about the fact that the union no longer has the support of the employees, they should be informed of their right to petition the National Labor Relations Board (NLRB) for decertification of the union, as stipulated in Section 9(c) of the National Labor Relations Act (NLRA). Upon request, a supervisor may tell employees that the necessary form may be obtained by any individual or group of employees from the NLRB regional office. Under no circumstances should a manager obtain the form for employees.

Recent case law has modified what employers are permitted to do. In *R.L. White Co., Inc.*, 262 NLRB No. 69, 111 LRRM 1078 (1982), the Board ruled that a company vice president could explain to employees how to have their union cards returned to them where the employer did not attempt to monitor whether employees would actually revoke their authorization cards and assures them that revocation is their decision. The Board said,

> An employer may lawfully inform the employees of their right to revoke their authorization cards, *even where employees have not solicited such information,* as long as the employer makes no attempt to ascertain whether employees will avail themselves of this right nor offers any assistance or otherwise creates a situation where employees would tend to feel in peril in refraining from such revocation. (Emphasis Added)

Even though this case involved only the revocation of union authorization cards, the principle seems to be applicable to the provision of *unsolicited* information to employees about their rights in decertifying the union. A bulletin board notice was utilized in one setting, for example (Exhibit 7–1). It is clear, however, that hospitals should discuss any such matters with a qualified labor attorney who stays informed on recent case law.

Employees should realize that at least 30 percent of the employees in the bargaining unit must sign the petition, or the petition will be dismissed and the union warned about the need to shore up its efforts. Decertification attempts are most commonly successful when the majority of employees have signed the

Exhibit 7–1 Letter to Employees on Union Decertification

TO: All Nursing Staff Employees

DATE:

A number of individuals have asked me how they could remove the Retail, Wholesale, Department Store Union, District 1199, as they no longer want the union to represent them. As I told them I would, I have contacted our attorney. He has advised me that if you, the employees, decide of your own individual free will that you do not want the RWDSU, District 1199 to represent you, you have the right to do the following:

> You may notify the hospital, *in writing and dated,* through a petition or other written statement that you do not want the union to represent you, and the hospital can then take the appropriate action if a *majority* of you, the employees, desire us to do so.

As I also informed them, the hospital is not inviting or urging you to sign any such petition, as it will make no difference in your working conditions. This decision is entirely up to you. Also, the hospital *will not* assist you in drafting or circulating such a petition, and such a petition or letter must not be circulated during your actual working time. It can be circulated only during breaks or lunch, or before or after work.

The law says that you are not required to have a union representing you if you do not wish to be represented by that union. Whether you want the union to represent you will make no difference in your treatment by the hospital.

The hospital simply wants to answer the questions you have raised so that you know and understand your rights.

                                       Good Samaritan Hospital

                                       John Doe, President

---

decertification petition. In brief, the petitioning effort should be made only when there is sufficient strength among employees.

Timing of a Decertification Petition

Intricate rules apply in selecting the proper time for filing the decertification petition. These rules include (1) the twelve-month rule, (2) the certification year rule, and (3) the contract bar rule.

The Twelve-Month Rule. A decertification election cannot be mandated when there has been a valid election during the preceding twelve-month period. The NLRB will process a petition filed within sixty days of the first anniversary of the valid election, however, and will schedule the election after the anniversary. Petitions filed prior to this sixty-day period are dismissed.

The Certification Year Rule. When a union receives NLRB certification, the majority status of the union must be recognized for one year, even if the union loses majority support in that year. In one situation, for example, the union promised benefits and scheduling changes, but never delivered them after the election. In anger, three months after the election, *all* the employees signed a decertification petition; their petition was not processed, however, because of the certification year rule.

When the union has a majority status as a result of voluntary recognition, i.e., there was no election, the hospital is obligated to recognize and bargain with the union for a reasonable period of time. The reasonable time frame is typically six months to one year.

The Contract Bar Rule. No decertification petition can be processed for the duration of a valid, executed contract lasting three years or less. Contractual agreements of longer than three years guarantee freedom from decertification petitions for the first three years.

When a contract is in effect, there are two options for filing a decertification petition. First, a petition may be filed during the "open period" of more than 90 but not over 120 days before the terminal date of a collective bargaining agreement involving a health care institution, under the rules as set out in *Trinity Lutheran Hospital,* 218 NLRB 199, 89 LRRM 1238 (1975). No petition is considered if filed within 90 days of contract termination, the "insulated period," so that the union and the hospital may negotiate without the pressure of an impending election. Second, the NLRB will accept a petition after the contract has expired.

Duty to Bargain

Until recently, in accordance with the NLRB's decision in *Telautograph Corporation,* 199 NLRB 892 (1972), employers could refuse to bargain when a decertification petition had been filed. In *Dresser Industries, Inc.,* 264 NLRB 145 (1982), the Board set aside the *Telautograph* decision, stating that the mere filing with the NLRB of a decertification petition is not grounds for a refusal to bargain. However, if the employer has evidence that a majority of employees signed the petition, if it is not during the certification year, and if there is no contract bar, the employer may withdraw recognition. Evidence of a majority is the decertification petition itself, if signed by a majority of employees, or an informal petition signed and dated by a majority of the employees involved, simply stating "We do not want to be represented by the union anymore." Of course, the employer cannot initiate, urge, circulate, sponsor, or in any way assist or promise benefits if the employees sign such a petition.

The Bargaining Unit

Determining the makeup of the bargaining unit is a vital step in the decertification process. In general, the bargaining unit is either the one *certified* or the one *recognized* by both parties. For example, dietary staff may have been certified originally as the bargaining unit, but members of the housekeeping staff, laboratory technicians, and licensed practical nurses may have been added to the unit over the years. Thus, the recognized unit differs from that originally certified.

When a multiple hospital system is recognized as a single bargaining unit, a labor attorney must investigate the collective bargaining history, as well as the actual composition of the unit involved and the unique circumstances of the involved parties, in order to determine what is the appropriate unit to decertify the union. While there is a landmark case based on bargaining history between the parties in which different plants are treated as a single unit (*General Electric Co.*, 180 NLRB 1094 [1970]), there are exceptions to the rule (e.g., *Duke Power Co.*, 191 NLRB 308 [1971]; *Mission Appliance Corp.*, 129 NLRB 1417 [1961]; *Clohecy Collision, Inc.*, 176 NLRB 616 [1969]).

While the union and the company may negotiate about the rights of particular voters, the bargaining unit is not larger than the one stipulated in the last bargaining agreement. As in other elections, votes may be challenged by the union. Successfully challenged votes may be the difference between winning and losing the decertification election.

When a strike is in effect at the time the decertification petition is filed, striking workers may have been permanently replaced in their jobs. Both the strikers and their replacements have the right to vote when an election is held within one year of the start of the strike. If 200 hospital employees went out on an economic strike and were permanently replaced, if decertification petition was signed, and if an election was held, a majority of 400 total employees eligible and/or 201 signatures would be needed for the decertification petition if it took place within one year of when the strike began. In the actual decertification election, the employer needs to have only a tie vote of those voting and the union still is decertified (*Best Motor Lines*, 82 NLRB 269 (1949)).

Deauthorization Petition

The purpose of a deauthorization petition is to cancel the requirement that all employees join the union where a union security clause is in force. This action is rare, but such a petition may be filed when the union fails to deliver on promises made during the organizing campaign. As in the decertification procedure, 30 percent of the employees must indicate interest by signing the petition. While winning the election pursuant to the deauthorization petition is effective in registering employee dissatisfaction, it does not remove the union as the collective bargaining agent for the employees.

Maintenance of membership provisions and other union security clauses founded on Section 8(a)(3) of the NLRA are subject to deauthorization petitions.

Election Procedure

The right to have a deauthorization election is based on Section 9(c) of the NLRA. The contract bar rule would not be applicable in such a case, since a contract with a union security clause must exist to make deauthorization proceedings a viable option. The deauthorization election is different from the other NLRB elections in that the petitioner must obtain the votes of a majority of those *eligible* to vote, not just a majority of the votes *cast,* to deauthorize the union.

Rationale for Deauthorization

When the employees win the deauthorization election, they have effectively relieved themselves of requirements inherent in the union security clause and are free to exercise their rights as stated in Section 7 of the NLRA by resigning from the union. Such an action on the part of the employees cannot have disciplinary repercussions that affect job status. Employees must withdraw from the union in writing (see *Struthers-Dunn, Inc.,* 228 NLRB 49 [1977]).

A deauthorization affects union income. Unless a hospital is a union shop, new employees are not required to join the union after thirty days of employment, and the union is unable to discipline members by imposing fines. Although the union is still responsible for collective bargaining and for enforcement of the contract, it cannot require membership or dues. In this situation, the union often loses interest in the needs of individuals in the bargaining unit. Mounting employee dissatisfaction with union service may result in a decertification proceeding at the end of the contract, as stipulated by rules for appropriate filing of a decertification petition.

Dues Checkoff

Administrators must be aware of the implications of dues checkoff authorizations. Section 302 of the Labor-Management Relations Act of 1947 defines the deduction of dues and other uniform payments that employers must pay to unions. Unions push hard to have a dues checkoff clause included in the contract so that the employer will be responsible for collecting union dues and paying them to the union.

In the right-to-work states, an agency shop may be permitted where the employee does not have to join but must pay a service fee and the dues checkoff is also a form of union security clause permitted. While such a contractual clause does not force an employee to sign a checkoff authorization as a condition of employment in these states, it does require the employer to honor the checkoff authorizations signed by its employees. Employees who sign checkoff authorizations usually have an escape period in which they have a right to change their minds. This employee right, as well as others related to authorization for checkoff, must be respected by both the union and the hospital. Failure to do so may result in an unfair labor practice charge.

An affirmative deauthorization vote enables employees to revoke the checkoff authorization, even though the terms of the authorization prohibit this (Exhibit 7-2). The NLRB has held in *Penn Cork & Closures, Inc.*, 156 NLRB No. 411 (1966), that, when there has been an affirmative deauthorization vote, outstanding checkoff authorizations originally executed by employees while a union-shop clause was in effect become vulnerable to revocation by employees "regardless of their terms" (156 NLRB No. 411, at 414-415). This is based on the fact that an election in which employees voted to deauthorize a union shop would be a "Pyrrhic victory" if employees were not allowed to stop paying union dues by revoking the dues checkoff authorizations. The employer must continue to collect dues, as required by any contractual requirement, and send them to the union until an employee has properly revoked the checkoff authorization card, however. *Bedford Can Manufacturing Corp.*, 162 NLRB No. 133 (1967).

Many employees do not understand their right to revoke their checkoff authorization cards during legally sanctioned time periods. Employers must walk a fine line when they inform employees about the facts of the checkoff authorization that they have signed. The NLRB has ruled that employers may inform employees of the revocability period and the automatic renewal features of a checkoff authorization. In *Perkins Machine Co.*, 141 NLRB 697 (1963), the Board upheld the employer's right to remind employees of their freedom to withdraw their authorizations by sending an unsolicited letter to employees' homes. In *Cyclops Corp.*, 216 NLRB 857 (1975), the Board found that paycheck reminders and a letter sent to the employees' homes after some employees had requested information was appropriate. It is imperative, however, that employers avoid checking on the subsequent

---

Exhibit 7–2 Checkoff Authorization

TO: Good Samaritan Hospital   DATE:

You are hereby authorized and directed to checkoff the designated dues (including initiation fee, if payable), starting with the first pay following your receipt of this authorization. The amount deducted shall be remitted by you to the Financial Secretary of District 1199, Retail, Wholesale, Department Store Union at ___[address]___, not later than the first day of the month following the month in which deductions were made.

This authorization is irrevocable for a period of one year from the execution hereof or until the termination date of the applicable collective bargaining agreement, whichever occurs sooner, and shall be automatically renewed for successive periods of one year or for the period of each succeeding applicable collective bargaining agreement, whichever period shall be shorter, unless written notice of its revocation by registered mail to the hospital and to the union is given by me fifteen days prior to any such renewal date.

_____
[Employee Signature]

action of employees in regard to these reminders. Such employer follow-up could be construed as a violation of Section 8 (a) (1) of the NLRA.

The union security and dues checkoff clauses terminate with termination of the collective bargaining agreement. When the new contract is signed, however, the authorizations will be automatically renewed by their own terms unless they were properly revoked.

Employer Petition

While it is not legal for an employer to sponsor, influence, or assist employees in making a decision to deauthorize or decertify the union, an employer may legally file a petition if there are facts to believe that the union has lost majority support. Such a petition, which must be supported by objective criteria, such as an employee petition, oral statements, or other valid facts from a majority of the employees, may be filed after the certification year is over and is valid as long as it is filed in an environment free of employer unfair labor practices. If there is a reasonable doubt supported by objective criteria as to the majority status of the union, the NLRB holds an election in which the union is required to reestablish its majority status.

At times, incumbent unions may merge or affiliate with another union. When such an action obscures the identity of the bargaining agent, the employer may file a petition to resolve the majority status of the new union representative under Board-sanctioned procedures or may refuse to bargain with the new representative so that the problem can be resolved in the subsequent defense of charges filed by the union.

A rival union may file an RC petition (simply an NLRB election petition filed by the union) to determine if employees wish to continue being represented by the incumbent union. Rules of timing, the election, and the 30 percent show of interest prevail in this case, as in the other types of elections. If the majority of employees vote to have no union, the hospital has no obligation to bargain with any collective bargaining agent. If there is no clear majority for the hospital, the incumbent union, or the rival union, there is a runoff election between the two receiving the most votes. It must be remembered that any attempt on the part of the employer to assist, solicit, or encourage attempts of the rival union are violations of the NLRA.

Finally, there is a UC petition (a unit clarification petition) by which supervisors or other groups of employees who are no longer considered part of an appropriate unit can be decertified from a unit. Such a petition should be filed when the old contract has lapsed and a new one has not yet been executed, however, it may also be filed when a contract is still in effect usually upon changed circumstances in the facts or the law.

In the Supreme Court case of *Beasley v. Food Fair, Inc.,* 416 U.S. 653 (1974), the right of the employer to discharge supervisors because of their union membership was upheld. This case underscores the prevailing policy covered by the NLRA that administrators are not expected to treat management personnel as employees, a policy opposed by some state nurses' organizations that represent all nurses, including supervisors. Hospitals should be aware of the law and the position of their state nurses' association on this issue. In summary, a successful withdrawal of union recognition comes only when a hospital is well prepared and equipped with a long-term action plan that takes into consideration strikes, permanent replacements for the strikers, and avoidance of unfair labor practices in the process always showing an intent to reach an agreement at the bargaining table that is fair and equitable to all.

MANAGEMENT AID IN THE DECERTIFICATION PROCESS

As mentioned earlier, an employer may not initiate, urge, or sponsor a decertification petition or deauthorization petition, but an employer may provide employees with the information required to make their own decision. Such information may be made available to employees in a question-answer format, even when they have not made specific inquiries about the deunionization process. The key is to ensure that the information provided on employee rights under the law is factual. When such information is made available in employee lounges or through some other routine method, the employer may not follow up in any way. *S.S. Kresge Co.*, Case No. 7-CA-1320, 7-CA-13170(2) (1976); *Woolco Department Store* 6024, 30-RD-402, 30-RM-361 (1977)[4] are two decisions which uphold an employer's right to provide employees with answers on the decertification process.

Although the employer may answer questions that employees have regarding their rights and the mechanism for revocation of checkoff authorization, deauthorization, or decertification, the employer must not render substantial aid. The employer may, however, render ministerial aid, defined as minor clerical, mechanical, or administrative assistance. For example, soliciting employees to file a decertification petition is substantial aid (illegal), whereas providing employees with factual information on the process is ministerial aid (legal). Employees are not allowed, legally, to pass around a deunionization petition during working hours, to use hospital equipment for the petition, or to seek hospital assistance. Also, hospital stationery should not be used for a decertification petition. While one of these practices may not constitute a case of substantial aid, several together might add up to unlawful assistance.

An employer may not write the decertification petition, but may discuss what employees might say in such a document. Likewise, letters of withdrawal from the union may not be written by the hospital, but management may make a sample letter of resignation available to employees upon request.

When the employer provides addresses, procedures, and other information helpful to employees in deunionization proceedings, the NLRB tends to find the conduct lawful, unless there have been unfair labor practices. Another point that is often examined in these cases is the equitable application of the no solicitation rule to all parties. The Board examines each case on its own merits and in great detail.

CAMPAIGNING IN DEUNIONIZATION PROCEEDINGS

There are some differences between a union organizing campaign (see Chapter 3) and a deunionization campaign. In the latter, employees have had experience with the union and are congregated around specific issues. When structuring communications to the staff in a decertification campaign, management should determine why the employees believed that the union was necessary and what has been changed or what the union has failed to deliver. In such an election, furthermore, employees must be made aware that in the voting procedure a vote of "No" means that they favor decertification, while a vote of "Yes" means that they want to retain their current union status.

Management must take great care not to connect any changes in wages, hours, or working conditions to the decertification process. If any hint of these changes is made in connection with employer threats or rewards, the union may file a charge with the NLRB thereby potentially compromising the current decertification efforts.

In a representation election, "buying time" is often the best strategy for the hospital. In a decertification or deauthorization election, however, it is to the union's advantage to stall, since time has a way of eroding the enthusiasm employees felt when they signed the petition. Therefore, hospital management should seek to have the decertification election as soon as possible.

The union may use several techniques to block the movement of the deunionization process. The union may file a "blocking charge" with the Board to halt the processing of the petition. The blocking charge is a term used by the NLRB to convey their policy to halt an election proceeding including a decertification election proceeding, because there is wrongful conduct being charged against one party which they claim interferes with the employee's free choice. The employer may counteract this charge by seeking injunctive relief in federal district court on the ground that the blocking charge prohibits employees from deciding for themselves whether they want the union to represent them. The following cases are illustrative of an employer going into federal district court claiming that the NLRB's administration of its blocking charge policy is illegally depriving the employees of their right: *Templeton v. Dixie Color Reprinting Co., Inc.*, 444 F.2d 1064, 77 LRRM 2392 (CA 5, 1971), vac'g and reman'g 74 LRRM 2206, 2319; *Surrat v. NLRB*, 463 F.2d 378, 80 LRRM 2804 (CA 5, 1972) aff'g 78 LRRM

2115.[5] Thus, it is crucial for an employer to minimize as much as possible giving the union opportunities to file unfair labor practice charges to set the NLRB's blocking charge policy in motion. Since these charges are usually claiming that the hospital is engaging in bad faith bargaining in order to create a strike to permanently replace the present employees, the employer must be very careful in the bargaining process. Preparation for a defense should include typewritten minutes of negotiations, as well as certified letters confirming all details of meetings, and reasons for failure to have meetings. Also, proposals with all concessions and the reasons that the hospital will not agree to certain proposals should be documented in writing.

When more than one union is fighting to represent the employees, the unions may make misstatements about each other. The employer with an effective communication network for disseminating information to employees can correct these misstatements. Written and verbal communications can restate union statements, inform employees of the truth, and state the employer's position on these statements.

When the decertification petition is filed during a strike, striker replacements may vote only in an economic strike. If the economic strike has gone beyond one year, the replaced strikers are not eligible to vote; only the striker replacements are eligible to vote. If surface bargaining (merely going through the motions with no intent to reach an agreement) is occurring at the bargaining table, the union may charge that the strike is not an economic one but an unfair labor practice strike and may successfully challenge the validity of votes cast in an election.

In some instances, unions have expelled members as a means of threatening others about job security. Employees need to be informed that they cannot lose their jobs in attempting to decertify the union, even when a union security clause is in effect, because they have been expelled from the union. The employer is not required to discharge an expelled employee except for nonpayment of dues if a union security clause is part of the contract. The hospital can use this union action to its own advantage by pointing out the facts of the situation and by showing the union's undemocratic tactics and its fear of an election.

Unions may also resort to fining members who support a decertification petition. Employers should advise employees who are threatened with such fines that fines based on the filing of decertification petitions or on the statutory right to refrain from union activity are not legal (*NLRB v. Molders, Local 125*, 442 F.2d 92 (CA 7, 1971), enforcing NLRB order at 178 NLRB 208 1969). Of course, the union may expel an individual who seeks decertification of it, see *Tawas Tube Products, Inc.*, 151 NLRB 46 (1965), but this will not affect their continued employment as long as they continue to offer to pay dues even under a union-shop clause. Employees who are fined for this reason may seek assistance from the NLRB in filing the appropriate charge. The hospital and other employees may also file charges about the illegal fining of a union member.

When a decertification attempt is being made, employers should inform their unionized employees that they can escape all union discipline by simply resigning in writing from the union on the day the union receives its written notice of the decertification petition. Resignation may not free employees from dues-paying obligations already incurred, but it does prevent the union from imposing fines.

After the hospital has met with employees, the union may request equal time for a speech on hospital property. An employer does not have to grant the union time and a place to meet with employees, however.

Unions sometimes threaten employees involved in a decertification campaign with violence. An unfair labor practice charge can be filed with the NLRB over such conduct, but such a charge stalls the processing of the decertification petition unless the employer files what is known as a "request to proceed" which merely means that although the employer has filed a charge that the union has coerced its employees, it still wants to proceed to the election at this time.

In summary, deunionization is only possible and feasible where a majority of the employees truly do not want the union to represent them. This must come from the employees as a ground swell without employer urging. The most fashionable way that deunionization is being accomplished in the 1980s is for employers to bargain tough over necessary management goals while attempting to gain employee support of its goals and preparing to take the inevitable strike. Deunionization then takes the turn of employees striking and the employer permanently replacing the striking employees. The permanent replacements then push decertification as the union is representing the replaced strikers whose only interests at this point are to force the employer to discharge the replacements. This is the most common form of deunionization today.

NOTES

1. William E. Fulmer, "When Employees Want to Oust Their Union," *Harvard Business Review,* 56 (March–April 1978): 163–171.

2. Franklin A. Shaffer, "The Decertification Process," *The Journal for Nursing Leadership and Management* 11 (September 1980): 55–47.

3. Benjamin Taylor and Fred Witney, *Labor Relations Law,* 4th ed. (Englewood Cliffs, NJ: Prentice-Hall, 1983).

4. Alfred T. DeMaria, *The Process of Deunionization* (New York: Executive Enterprises Publications, 1979).

5. Ibid.

Part II

Contemporary Problems

Chapter 8

The Communications Network

Communications is probably the most critical area of concern to managers who are working to effect an excellent employee relations program. When management loses its credibility and its ability to talk to its employees effectively, unionization is not far behind. Employees are influenced by their own belief systems, as well as by those of the group to which they belong as employees at a hospital. An awareness of current employee attitudes, opinions, complaints, and comments is crucial for equitable and appropriate management policies and actions.

The communication network in an institution is like the nervous system in the human body. Effective communication begins with sensors that detect problems, issues, and concerns at the grass roots of the organization. When information is received at this level, managers must compare it with other input. After the message has been interpreted, it is conveyed in upward, lateral, and downward channels of communication among group members and to related subgroups. Thus, higher level management learns about group responsibility, achievements, and productivity from the middle manager representing the employee group. At the same time, the manager establishes effective communications to keep the employee group functioning like a team. Dysfunction at any point may cause localized problems or major disturbances that influence functional operations of the entire system.

An effective communication network includes a mechanism for identifying and telling employees what they need to know, what they want to know, techniques to promote communication in all directions, and methods of evaluating the effectiveness of the network.

SURVEYS OF EMPLOYEE NEEDS

Managers have often been quite surprised to learn how different employee priorities are from management estimates of those priorities.[1] One of the best ways to learn about employee needs and problems in specific areas is an organizational survey. Such a survey also provides a systematic, anonymous method of determining the effectiveness of management strategies. These may be standardized surveys that reflect national norms, or they may be tailor-made to fit the particular needs of an individual hospital. Many surveys also include an open-ended answer section in which employees can add their personal comments. In these surveys, employees may be asked about work organization, work efficiency, administrative effectiveness, leadership practices, communications, personnel policies and procedures, satisfaction with patient care standards, pay and benefits, immediate supervision, work associates, job satisfaction, organizational identification and competitiveness, advancement opportunities, and job security.

After analyzing the survey to identify key problems and needs, managers can work to gather more information on the causes of problems. The problem-solving method is a useful approach in this process. The project should end with recommendations and planned action for necessary changes or shifts in emphasis. To ensure that the project is utilized, managers should specifically delineate who is to follow up, as well as how and when such follow-up action can be expected.

Managers may wish to do an informal, anonymous survey by asking a group of employees to rank a list of items such as the following from most to least important.

- good wages and fringe benefits
- job security
- feeling "in" on things
- sympathetic help on personal problems
- full appreciation of work
- tactful disciplining
- personal loyalty to workers
- promotion and growth in the organization
- work that keeps you interested
- good working conditions

Managers should rank the list as they think their employees will, rather than using the list to gauge the manager's sentiments. In this way, the results of the employee group can be compared with the results of management.

In one survey based on similar items, employees expressed a desire to know that the organization was modern and competitive in the market, as they considered these factors important in their own job security. Raises and benefits were the next most significant to the group because of the state of the economy. In the area of self-esteem and recognition, the employees felt that it was important to know that the organization valued their efforts and contributions. The employees also wanted to feel informed about hospital business; they expressed embarrassment at seeing news in the newspaper first. The majority of the group emphasized that they could tolerate many adverse conditions, if only the supervisors would be fair in treatment and discipline of all employees, and would show appreciation for employees' hard work. The nurses in the group stressed the importance of being able to share in the decision-making process in patient care and in unit work patterns.

Most of the comments in the open-ended portion of the survey related to people irritations such as

- "The supervisor corrects employees in the hall right in front of everyone."
- "Some people get whatever shifts they want. If they are absent, no one seems to correct them. If I did some of those things, I would be fired."
- "The linens never come up to the floor in time to give baths."
- "The newspaper story told me that my wing was closing before I heard it from my head nurse."
- "Administration is always promising us more help, but they never come through with someone who actually knows what they are doing enough to really help us."
- "I would like to sit down with the head administrator and have a gripe session."
- "My head nurse would take it out on me if I told administration what was really going on up here."
- "The administrators don't understand how much sicker the patients are today than they have ever been before. I run my tail off when I work."

Clearly, the results of the survey and the open forum indicated deeply rooted problems at the hospital. The administrators worked hard to institute a sound communications program in which employee needs were a top priority. Within four months, employees were expressing positive thoughts and the turnover at the hospital had been cut by 30 percent.

MANAGERIAL PROBLEMS IN COMMUNICATING

There are so many competing stimuli in the hospital environment that the importance of communication and recognition of employees is often overlooked. Meantime, employees grow increasingly upset at management's failure to acknowledge their efforts. Managers sometimes say that employees know they are appreciated without verbal reinforcement, but this is not the case—employees do not read minds. The *only* way to know what employees really think is to stay in constant touch with them and ask them for their input.

Managers have more pragmatic problems in communicating with employees as well. Sometimes the managerial group is given information that, if it became known, could bring adverse publicity on the hospital or compromise its position with competitors. If this information leaks to employees' their managers should not criticize top management, but should take a positive view of the situation. The manager might say to employees, "Being in a competitive position with other hospitals sometimes means that only a few people can know what is going on. They need to strike while the iron is hot and the politics are right. Taking time to tell all of us could mean that they lose their competitive edge. As long as our leaders are making solid plans for our future, we should feel good. If others get into the paper and we don't, we need to start worrying." At the same time, the management team needs to ensure that employees do receive information and that employees' opinions are requested in less critical matters. The underlying principle in communications must be to develop a trusting relationship with employees.

Many managers find their attempts to communicate with employees frustrating. Exhibit 8-1 contains a summary of effective human relations techniques.

COMPLAINTS

Employees want to be heard and to see action when they pass on complaints or suggestions to management. Many times a request for a system to handle complaints is really a request for an effective upward, downward, and lateral communication network.

Objectives

Effective complaint systems achieve the following objectives: (1) they get to the message or feelings underlying the complaint, (2) they are readily used by employees, and (3) they maintain good employee and supervisory morale. To achieve the first objective, managers must have their fingers on the pulse of the organization. If they know what is happening and who makes it happen, they are in a good position to interpret complaints with a realistic perspective. To encourage employee use of the system, managers must make the system credible, responsive, and safe to users. Employees will not use the complaint mechanism if doing so brings the wrath of supervisors down upon them.

The administrator must ensure that supervisors understand the importance of a workable complaint system and do not feel threatened by it. Supervisors need to be aware of the mouse-for-an-elephant theory; sometimes a small concession in the near future can bring long-term benefits on more significant issues. Furthermore,

Exhibit 8–1 Ten Commandments of Human Relations

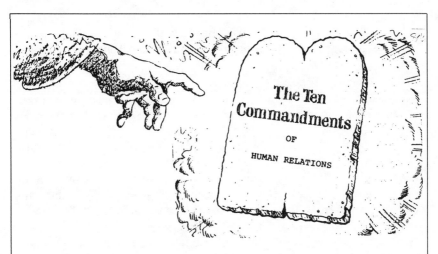

1. Listen to your employees. Hear them out whether the problem is "real" or "imagined." Know their interests and needs.
2. Recognize your employees. Everyone likes praise for a job well-done. Resolve all complaints promptly.
3. Talk to all of your employees regularly.
4. Be up front. Tell the good with the bad. If you criticize an employee, tell him or her how to correct the problem.
5. Keep all your employees well-informed. Encourage suggestions and follow-up.
6. Be sincere and honest with your employees. Show warm human concern in your employees' problems.
7. Take an interest in your employees' feelings, talents, and significant events.
8. Be fair, reliable, and friendly.
9. If the above produces no results, be firm and consistent. never go back on your word.
10. Keep the golden rule: Do unto others as you would have them do unto you.

employees will not use a system in which the supervisors are always supported, regardless of the facts in the situation. Supervisors need to view give and take as more important than unwavering rightness.

Open Door Policy

When the open door policy works well, it can be a major deterrent to unionization and an effective way to handle complaints. Managers who listen sincerely to employees and take action that is best for employees should be able to get beneath surface demands to the real issues of personal and financial well-being, confidence in management, and the needs for fair and equal treatment.

There are five key ingredients in a workable open door system for complaints:

1. Advertise it. Employees can be informed that an open door complaint system exists through personal encounters, memos, bulletin boards, meetings, and the hospital newspaper.
2. Be available. If possible, managers should be available when the shift changes to handle simple, drop-in complaints. If a spontaneous meeting is not possible, a definite appointment time should be scheduled within one day of the employee request. In addition to meeting with employees about complaints, it is helpful for top managers to be visible to greet employees informally.
3. Get all the facts. When meeting with an employee about a complaint, it is essential for the manager to allow the employee to explain the problem fully from a personal perspective. Then the manager should tell the employee what additional information is required before a decision on the matter can be made and approximately how much time this additional data collection will require. After the employee has gone, the manager can use a variety of resources to obtain the necessary facts, such as interviews with appropriate others, referral to the policy book, investigation into similar cases, input from opinion surveys, and data from exit interviews.
4. Keep the employee posted. When the necessary information has been gathered, the manager should give the employee some type of status report to indicate that the matter is not being dropped. If the manager decides not to make any changes because the employee solution is incompatible with departmental or institutional objectives, the employee should be told about that decision and allowed to discuss alternative actions. Employees must feel confident that their requests are taken seriously.
5. React appropriately. Demonstrate to employees that all complaints and suggestions receive honest attention. No one likes a listener who nods politely, but fails to act appropriately.

There are several key points to remember in using an open door system:

1. Managers must phrase points in terms of *what* is right, rather than in terms of *who* is right so that the discussion does not turn into a blame-setting session in which the issues are not fully explored because of one party's defensiveness.
2. Managers must stick to the facts and gear the discussion away from emotionally charged words that bog down progress.
3. Managers should admit mistakes. Credibility is greatly enhanced when managers feel comfortable in saying, "I goofed!" or "I don't know, but I will find out."

4. When an open door policy program is new, the first complaints are often intended to "test the water." The correct handling of these complaints is essential to the success of the open door effort.
5. Managers should take all complaints seriously. What may seem trivial to the manager is often very important to the employee. The seemingly insignificant personal conflicts and irritations are often the items that bother people the most on a job.
6. Employees should not be required to justify their complaints. Instead, managers should focus on their interest on resolving the problem.
7. Managers must listen carefully to what the employee is saying to hear the real or imagined problem that underlies the complaint. It is often not *what* was done, but *how* it was done.
8. When an apology is required, managers should apologize sincerely.
9. Managers need not have all of the answers or pretend to have ultimate authority. They should be honest when they require more authority or information to work on the problem. Employees probably already know the limits of a manager's authority.

For a summary of important points in handling complaints, see Exhibit 8–2.

CONFLICT RESOLUTION

Conflict is not always negative; it can be positive or neutral. In a hospital, however, conflict can turn into big problems when it is not acknowledged and dealt with openly. It is important for hospital managers to answer the following three questions:

1. How does conflict arise in the work setting?
2. Is conflict encouraged or discouraged?
3. How are individuals coping with conflict as it exists in the hospital?

After answering these questions, managers should ask themselves what can be done to improve conflict resolution in the future.

A hospital system is comprised of interdependent parts. One type of conflict arises when scarce or undistributable goods are not available to satisfy the needs and values of all parts of the system. Conflict may also arise because needs vary among the various parts of a system. For instance, in one situation physicians were keeping the operating rooms filled with cases. Nurses were upset about the high patient census because they did not have the trained staff to give the proper care. Nurse-physician communications were becoming a full-blown cold war. Physicians were critical of the nurses when working with them and when speaking to

Exhibit 8–2 Supervisor's Checklist for Handling Complaints

1. Don't berate employee in front of fellow workers.
2. Allow the employee to tell his or her side of the story.
3. Get all the facts.
4. Write it down.
5. Don't blame the employee, but try and correct the problem in a friendly manner.
6. Does the employee feel he or she can go over your head, if needed?
7. Is this a case where you can give a mouse for an elephant?
8. Get at the real problem.
9. Don't come down on an employee because he or she goes over your head or files a complaint.

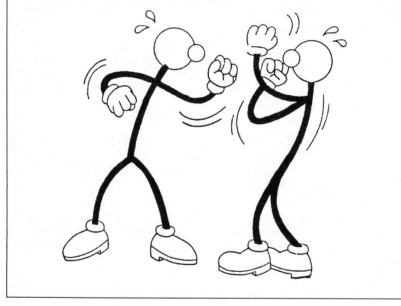

patients. Nurses felt that their hard work was going unnoticed and that no one understood their staffing needs. Management intervened by having nurse-physician problem-solving sessions to identify the elements of the problem. Because the physicians planned to keep the patient census high, nursing managers recruited seasoned nurses from other areas of lower demand. The surgical nurses worked with the managers to provide a solid orientation program that was condensed into two weeks. During this period, physicians relaxed their operating schedules. As a result of this collaboration, a serious conflict was successfully resolved.

Obstacles to Conflict Resolution

Noncommunication is one of the major obstacles to conflict resolution. Obviously, problems cannot be solved when involved persons are unwilling to verbalize the issues and work through the problem-solving process.

Sometimes people who are not directly involved in a conflict take sides. Then, communication of group members with certain other persons is viewed as an act of disloyalty to the group. Such a stance deflects the conflict from the issues to the personalities and frustrates efforts for resolution.

Scapegoating is also unproductive in conflict resolution because it displaces the conflict from a powerful party to one that is less powerful. For example, John just learned at a meeting with the administrator that an area he had been supervising for some time was being assigned to another assistant administrator, who was in better favor with the administrator. Because that area was the one in which the greatest hospital growth was anticipated, it guaranteed its supervisor more power in the hospital. After the meeting, John made his usual rounds to all of the areas he supervised, but he was short-tempered with employees. When one employee voiced dissatisfaction with staffing, he made a remark that undermined the efforts of top management. Thus, the conflict kept simmering and made problems in the other hospital areas supervised by John much worse.

Sometimes hospital managers believe that it is best to deny or suppress the conflict. Such an approach to the problem only allows the conflict to simmer and grow into greater proportions. Instead, managers must learn as much as possible about the conflict. Inadequate understanding or failure to collect enough data can keep managers from selecting approaches that are effective in conflict resolution.

In some hospitals conflict is readily apparent in the way employees relate to each other, managers relate to employees, and managers relate to each other. This negative work environment is commonly caused by a lack of trust. For example, in one unionized setting, the entire management team was meeting to determine the strategy for the approaching negotiations. These meetings seemed fruitless, however, and were characterized by a paucity of communication. The chief executive officer believed that the lack of communication resulted from the managers' lack of knowledge about labor relations; the truth was that managers were afraid to speak because they feared retaliation. When the problem of mistrust was exposed, most members of the group slowly affirmed the problem. Clearing the air was the first step in establishing the communication that the managers needed to function cohesively as a group. As they continued to meet, the group built a bond of trust and collaborated effectively on the issues that were facing them as managers.

Conflicts that are unrealistically assessed or interpreted are unlikely to be resolved. It is important to be open-minded when dealing with conflict so that all factors can be carefully evaluated. In establishing the climate for conflict resolution, managers must avoid giving the impression that other managers or employees need to be submissive in order to be virtuous. Retaliation on those who identify conflict can break down the bidirectional communication channels.

Goals in Conflict Resolution

A good decision must be based on all factors, including emotion. When emotion is recognized, expressed, and considered in management decisions, employees will accept and implement appropriate activity more wholeheartedly. When employment pressures require employees to disguise certain feelings and act in accord with those distortions, however, the result is conflict. Chronic resentment and anger heighten conflict, increase the occurrence of psychosomatic disorders, and lead to inappropriate displacement and eruptions. Such behaviors give poor corporate impressions on the public and on other professionals involved in the hospital.

The following goals are important considerations in successfully handling conflict:

1. Accept the complexity of human motivation and the intricacy of human egos to avoid oversimplification of the issues.
2. Recognize conflict as an opportunity for growth and learning.
3. Internalize all sides of the issues so that all points can be objectively assessed.
4. Visualize changes in values and in the current situation that are necessary to resolve the conflict most effectively and creatively.
5. Build flexibility within the system to allow for conflict resolutions that encourage growth.
6. Recognize that the means toward desired ends may themselves turn into primary drives.

COPING WITH ANONYMITY

There are no perfect answers to every problem in human relations, because humans themselves are imperfect. Since the beginning of time, however, organizations have strived to create the perfect system. When things do not fit their system, managers have tried to make them fit, experiencing constant frustration in working toward something that does not operate as smoothly as theoretically it should.

Hospitals need goals, philosophies, purposes, and people dedicated to programs that incorporate planned change and good management. Progress toward those programs is not evident in every behavior, however. For example, written goals do not always seem to affect the way that managers and employees operate on a daily basis, but they provide a touchstone for evaluating progress in the same hospital over time and among area competitors. Analysis of goals and programs can also tell administrators how the hospital stands in relation to the national leading health care institutions.

Typically, large organizations operate in what March and Cohen termed a "loosely coupled system."[2] In this system, many things are never communicated because of information overload, problems arising from politics of the institution, and the low priority of detail in communication if all is going well. When a part of the system breaks down, more attention is given to communication until the nonfunctional part returns to normal; then, the quantity of communication is reduced. After all, if everything in an institution were communicated to everyone, none of the institution's work would be done.[3,4]

Loosely coupled systems are characterized by a lack of specific goals for daily activity, limited supervision, and a loose feedback network. Basically, as long as everything is operating smoothly, the system allows its members to do their jobs with very little administrative interference. Thus, employees and managers generally enjoy a great deal of power, freedom, and autonomy. When something goes wrong, however, this system tightens up. For example, when it is determined that Susan Smith is a diabetic, she is admitted to the hospital. The pediatric team provide their usual excellent care and do the requisite teaching on the condition and its care to the child and family. Dr. Smith, her father and a very influential staff physician, complains about the quality of care, even though the problem is his failure to accept the disease in his daughter. Dr. Smith goes to the administrator, who "investigates" the problem with the nursing care. In this process, everything is questioned, people are asked about "the" way to provide care to a diabetic patient, and the usual flexibility disappears. In sum, the crisis caused the system of care on pediatrics to become a tightly coupled system, in which everything is rigid. Staff members are uncomfortable working in such a system, but they know that the system will return to its loosely coupled state when the crisis blows over.

Managers should be aware of certain characteristics of the loosely coupled system so that coping with day-to-day people problems becomes easier:

- Problematic preferences. Most people have flexible priorities; that is, the items that are most important to them are directly related to their experience and contemporary perceptual world.
- Unclear technology. There is no single way that is exclusively right in most situations.
- Fluid participation. Individuals in hospitals are not always equally involved in every decision because their interest and their ability to be physically present changes in every situation.

In the case of Susan Smith, for example, Dr. Smith's problematic preferences changed because of the illness of his daughter; previously, he had not been concerned about childhood diabetes. Now, however, he wanted clear-cut procedures for Susan's care. While there are some basic principles, these are modified to the needs of each patient and to the style of the nurse working with the child and family, i.e., the technology is unclear. Finally, the principle of fluid participation is seen in the fact that Dr. Smith had no input into decision making on pediatrics until his personal interest caused him to be continually present during the stay of his daughter.

While loosely coupled systems are relatively comfortable to work in, the authority in noncrisis situations is diffused so that obtaining a well-delineated answer to a specific problem can be difficult. Learning to live with gray answers to many questions is important for hospital managers, because they work in loosely coupled systems and in environments that mirror the rapid rate of change in society at large. They must find a system, such as the loosely coupled system, that assists them in rationally dealing with the operations of people-intensive systems. By maintaining a sense of humor and perspective and by working well with people, progress toward important hospital goals will be made over the long run.[5-7]

COMMUNICATION TECHNIQUES

Three techniques are particularly valuable in working effectively and communicating with employees. These include the open door policy discussed earlier, the communigram, and daily talks.

Sound Off Communigrams

The sound off program involves placing suggestion boxes at various points in the hospital so that employees can say what is on their minds, either personally or anonymously, by means of communigrams. The entire procedure for the sound off program includes a committee and a follow-up mechanism.

The program may be introduced to employees by an announcement with the actual communigram that will be placed around the hospital to read as follows:

> We are glad to hear your suggestions, ideas, concerns, and complaints at sound off. Do not feel that you have to justify your thoughts. You are encouraged to use the communigram to say what's on your mind, to make your suggestions, ideas, concerns, and complaints known informally (and anonymously if desired). Give us enough information to understand the situation. Describe it as much as possible so that the sound off committee will understand. Thank you for sharing your thoughts with us.
>
> 1. My suggestion/idea/concern/complaint is:
> 2. Remedy requested:
> 3. Problem avoidance:

All communigrams will be promptly handled by the sound off committee. Employees choosing to sign a communigram will receive an individual written reply.

Care must be taken in using the sound off program to avoid dominating or interfering with the formation or administration of a labor organization, a violation of Section 8(a)(2) of the NLRA (see *NLRB v. Ampex Corporation*, (CA-7) 442 F.2d 82 1971). In *Scott & Fetzer Co. (The Streamway Div.) v. NLRB*, (CA-6) 95 LC ¶ 13,810 (1982), however, an employee committee established by management to improve communications was held not to be a labor organization. The Sixth Circuit Court of Appeals reversed the holding of the NLRB that the company's establishment of such a committee was a violation of Section 8(a)(2) of the NLRA. The court found the NLRB's ruling that the employee committee was a "labor organization" to be an "overly broad" interpretation, holding that the ruling could thwart the purposes of the NLRA by preventing employees from conferring with management unless they form a union.

Principles of a Sound Off Program

One successful sound off program was as follows:

1. This effort is advertised so that employees feel they have a voice in their affairs.
2. A rotating committee is appointed; it is comprised of (1) the chief executive officer; (2) a physician representative; (3) two registered nurses; (4) one licensed practical nurse or aide; (5) the director of nursing; (6) a representative from housekeeping or maintenance; (7) a representative from occupational therapy, physical therapy, pharmacy, social service, laboratory, or radiology; and (8) a personnel representative as an ombudsperson. All members have one vote on issues. The chief executive officer has the right to break any ties in voting or to veto any decision that would not be in the best interests of the hospital.
3. All complaints must first be discussed with the employee's immediate supervisor and then may be brought before the committee. Complaints are not screened unless they invade the privacy of an individual. Complaints should specify the policy or procedure that is claimed to be violated.
4. The committee has the authority to ask any individual to present a factual account of a situation to the committee.
5. Minutes for all meetings are recorded and kept on file.
6. There is a deadline for a response to complaints or for corrective action to be taken.

7. If possible, corrective action is taken in at least one employee complaint a month.
8. A representative from personnel acts as an ombudsperson for an employee who wants to bring a complaint to the committee.
9. To facilitate the use of the complaint procedure and to avoid chilling anyone's ideas, suggestions, or complaints, Communigrams are provided throughout the hospital for filing anonymous complaints.
10. All answers to complaints become part of the formal minutes. Minutes should show all action taken.
11. In cases of indecision, the chief executive officer makes the final decision.
12. A quorum of the group consists of six members.
13. Any employees who file a complaint may have anyone from the hospital staff speak for them, if they so desire. If the committee does not want to have a particular individual speak for the employee who has the complaint, the committee may answer the complaint, with no further investigation, on the data available at that time.
14. Employees are selected for this committee by the chief executive officer.
15. The committee meets at least monthly.

The following questions should be covered by your hospital's sound off committee, if one is established:

1. Should a physician be on the committee?
2. Should minutes be taken at meetings?
3. Should employees be able to represent each other?
4. What kind of problems do you foresee in implementation of this idea?
5. Should there be timetables spelled out?

Daily Talks

In hospitals that have implemented the technique of daily talks, managers have noticed a vast improvement in their understanding of what is going on and in the response of employees to them. The usefulness of this program cannot be overemphasized.

Daily talks are brief messages to every front line supervisor from the director. The supervisors are then charged with the responsibility for relaying this information to their subordinates and encouraged to report feedback to the director. Employee feedback is utilized in making decisions, and employees are kept posted on how their input has been considered and used. In addition to providing information on required actions, the daily talks program can be used to pass on information of general interest to employees. This program gets supervisors into the habit of giving employees periodic briefings.

In one hospital, the chief executive officer was planning to add one more holiday to the benefit package. He asked supervisors to poll the employees to see what type of day they preferred. Responses from every department were kept and tallied. Supervisors were surprised at employees' enthusiasm in being asked to participate in decision making. Furthermore, while responding to the specific question of holidays, employees also had the opportunity for face-to-face communication about a myriad of other, unrelated concerns. Supervisors followed up on the unrelated items as well as on the specific request about holidays. Once the director got the feedback from the employees, results were tallied and communicated to the employees. A floating holiday was then added to the holiday benefit package, and the supervisors thanked employees for their input. Supervisors commented that they had not realized that their busy schedules kept them from speaking to employees more often. Moreover, the chief executive officer found that he gained feedback on many other issues, and he encouraged the use of this technique at least weekly in all departments.

In the nursing department, the director of nursing implemented the program further by holding a briefing session of fifteen minutes with supervisors on all three shifts twice weekly. This briefing did not take the place of executive meetings, but instead highlighted significant events that were occurring in the hospital. Supervisors felt better informed and were able to relay important communications to area coordinators and shift leaders for dissemination to the staff. Feedback to the director of nursing improved, as did her relationship with shift supervisors and coordinators. The nursing department began to operate more smoothly because of the improved communication among all members of the department. The success of this technique underscores the importance of recognizing the worth of every individual in the operation of the hospital.

Supplemental Techniques

Many other techniques help to improve communications with employees.

Quality Circles. A number of hospitals are experimenting with the concept of quality circles, a complex technique in which a group is assigned to work on a problem. Group members must be trained in the way that the hospital system works so that their efforts are both supported and consistent with other mechanisms available in the hospital. The group needs specific training in group process and in change, as well as administrative support for its activity. A liaison is needed to coordinate group efforts with other parts of the system. When the group arrives at a realistic solution to a problem, the system's commitment to the quality circles concept must be great enough to utilize the group input. If the work of the group is in vain, a morale problem can be created.[8-10]

Letters to Employees. Letters from the chief executive officer to employees can be used to discuss the information gleaned from opinion surveys, new regulations, statistics indicating growth, and efforts to implement the hospital philosophy. Possible letter themes include:

- the annual hospital picnic...
- compliments from our clients...
- thank you for your effort...
- absenteeism hurts you...
- new federal regulations...
- implementing our philosophy...
- growth plans for...
- new benefits...

Paycheck Inserts. Any time that an important bit of information should be conveyed to all employees, a paycheck insert may be considered. For example, if the hospital is being organized, a simulated checkoff as a paycheck insert can be used to show employees how much money they will be missing from their paychecks for union dues and initiation fees.

Employee Manuals. When new employees join the organization, they should be given an employee manual in a loose-leaf format. The last page should contain a statement to be signed by the employee indicating that he or she has read the contents of the manual and has had ample opportunity to ask questions about it. This sheet is removed from the manual and becomes a permanent part of the employee's record. Current employees should have access to the same information and to updated manual inserts as policies change. It may be wise to give a refresher orientation to employees who have been with the organization for a certain number of years so that employees have regular reviews of new policies. Such a refresher course does not negate employee responsibility for remaining up-to-date.

Telephone Anonymous. The hospital may also reach out to employees by providing a telephone line with a recorded message and a mechanism that employees can use to offer ideas, suggestions, and complaints anonymously.

Small Group Sessions. It is helpful for area leaders and top supervisors to meet periodically with employees in small groups to discuss and resolve issues and problems, as well as to share information.

Bulletin Boards. A very effective, inexpensive way to reach employees on a daily basis is to use a bulletin board. To get the maximum effect from bulletin boards, they should be placed where they can be read under relaxed circumstances.

Items should be brief and should be dated; they should be changed periodically. A specific person should be assigned to each board to monitor posted content and to keep the board in order. Bulletin boards can be developed on a theme, such as

- Management notices
- Hats off
- Did you know ...?
- Compliments from ...
- Briefs on new employees, with photos
- Lost and found
- Trading post
- Kudos
- Humor
- Health topic themes or safety
- Job opportunities
- New products or program trends
- Director's corner

Other bulletin boards can be designed for patient waiting areas.

House Publications. Like bulletin boards, a house publication can be extremely varied and creative. Since publications are often circulated to more than employees, however, they may not serve the complete needs of the staff for information. A separate publication, especially for employees, may be needed.

Rounds. There is nothing like a walking tour of the work area with the area manager, a staff nurse, and maybe someone who is being oriented. The apprenticeship method is a good way to learn the tricks of master clinicians. This valuable form of communication helps managers identify problems and provide on-the-spot feedback to those in attendance. Naturally, rounds can be used for several purposes, and those in attendance are determined by the purpose of the specific rounds.

Grapevine. An analysis of the news and views on the grapevine to determine key individuals, interrelationships in the organization, and ways that data may be effectively transmitted through the grapevine can be very helpful. Vital branches should be kept open so that news can be transmitted on it.

Retreat. Managers retreat for one or two days to discuss problems and design objectives to make the hospital more competitive.

Counseling. Employees should have a one-to-one meeting with their supervisor no less than biannually. At this time, individual concerns can be aired so that personal objectives and issues can be clarified.

Exit Interviews. People are especially candid and often feel that they need not hesitate to complain or suggest ideas when they are leaving a position. Therefore, managers can gain valuable information by analyzing exit interview data.

Show and Tell. In one hospital, employees compete in decorating their units for the year-end holidays. Prizes are given to the top three areas. In addition, everyone is encouraged at this time of year to take a few minutes over several days and visit other areas to learn what they are doing. Unfortunately, the bigger the hospital, the more difficult interunit communication can be.

Such interunit sharing can be the beginning of "Special Unit Spotlight" events, in which one unit may display its new programs and plans for all of the other units. Perhaps, this new knowledge about other areas will become the basis of nurse-to-nurse consultations. This effort meshes nicely with a cross-training program in which staff members work regularly on units that have similar needs.

Which One for Your Hospital?

Good communication does not just happen; it requires a great deal of effort. Managers should take the following steps to determine which approach is right for their hospital:

1. Formally and informally survey employee opinions.
2. Obtain input from all managers on the type of communication techniques that will work best for the hospital and its departments.
3. Develop a game plan that details how to improve communication in the hospital, how to evaluate the system, and how to implement your plan. Include deadlines and budget time and money to ensure successful implementation of the program.

NOTES

1. Ellen Joy Bernstein, "Employee Attitude Surveys: Perception vs. Reality," *Personnel Journal* 60 (April 1981): 300–305.

2. Cohen and March, *Leadership and Ambiguity: The American College President* (New York: McGraw-Hill, 1974).

3. George Kuh, "Using Alternative Organizational Perspectives in Student Affairs" (Indiana University, 1982, unpublished).

4. Joyce Riffer, "Pilot Program in Maine Hospital Shows How Nurses, Physicians Can Collaborate," *Hospitals* 55 (November 1981): 17–24.

5. Bernstein, "Employee Attitude Surveys."

6. Kuh, "Using Alternative Organizational Perspectives."

7. Riffer, "Pilot Program in Maine Hospital."

8. John Baird, "Quality Circles May Substantially Improve Hospital Employees' Morale," *Modern Healthcare* 11 (September 1981): 70, 72, 74.

9. Kenneth M. Jenkins and Justin Shimada, "Quality Circles in the Service Sector," *Supervisory Management* 1 (August 1981): 3–7.

10. Donald E. Johnson, "Quality Circles Put Workers in Charge of Their Productivity," *Modern Healthcare* 11 (September, 1981): 68–69,

Chapter 9

Discipline Is...

Discipline should be viewed as a broad concept. The stage for an effective disciplinary program is established by hiring practices, orientation, synchronization of job descriptions with performance appraisals and comparable worth, actual disciplinary procedures, and legislation affecting the health care industry specifically and the country in general.

HIRING PRACTICES

Laws on discrimination are complex, ambiguous, and constantly changing. Managers in health care institutions should subscribe to some type of service that keeps them up-to-date on the case law in this area to ensure that they are complying with the laws on hiring and firing. Moreover, any changes in pre- or postemployment requirements for employment should be validated with an attorney specializing in Equal Employment Opportunity (EEO) law.

Each question on an application or in an interview should be defensible on the basis of job-related information that will be utilized in a fair, unbiased manner to support employment decisions. Such questions should be job-related so that they can be justified as being asked for as a legitimate business necessity. In following good personnel practice in employment programs, managers should:

1. define skill requirements by a careful job analysis
2. make a special effort to recruit minorities
3. be certain that all screening and interviewing procedures are related to job requirements
4. validate any tests on the basis of job-related criteria and ensure that the test results can be correlated with job performance requirements and not discriminate against any protected class

5. be certain that any skill test is administered under proper conditions and in an objective manner that is validated and defensible
6. base all employment programs on the written policies and procedures governing the operation at the hospital

The organization charged with discrimination must validate its selection procedures in relation to the alleged discriminatory activity. When discrimination exists, so-called adverse impact can be shown in two ways. First, the adverse impact may be the outcome or result of facially neutral practices. Second, the procedure and practices leading to the adverse impact may be at fault. Thus, employers need to examine both the means and the end of their personnel practices.

Employment Screening

In general, the administrator involved in hiring must be guided by the principle that it is unlawful to make inquiries into matters relating to race, color, religion, sex, age, national origin, ancestry, or handicap, unless such inquiry can be supported as a BFOQ or job-related inquiry. Also no inquiry should be made about an applicant's former or current union activities.

In many hospitals today people such as head nurses have been given a great deal of discretion in hiring because of increasing decentralization and because of the hospital's desire to have them qualify as supervisors under the National Labor Relations Act (NLRA). While personnel interviewers are well aware of the legal restrictions on interviews, head nurses may not be aware of such restrictions. In all innocence a head nurse may ask questions about an applicant's transportation to work, parental responsibilities, and nationality or language capacities that violate the law. The head nurse may also make innocent inquiries into experience with the American Nurses' Association (ANA) or other unions. Forewarned is forearmed.

Name. An applicant may be asked to state his or her full name. It is lawful to ask the applicant for name changes, nicknames, or other identification under which previously employed that allows the employer to check work references or educational records.

Address. Managers may ask applicants to state their address, along with their length of residence. Applicants may also be asked to list prior addresses and the length of time they lived at each address. Specific inquiry into foreign addresses is not advised unless it is a BFOQ or is job-related.

Sex. To be a part of the application, sex must be established as a BFOQ or job-related item. Most people eliminate the question and merely ask the receptionist to note the race and sex for reasons of keeping applicant flow statistics so that good faith efforts to employ minorities can be shown. The record the receptionist keeps is called the EEO-1 job applicant log.

Religion/Creed. Only if it is a BFOQ or job-related item can an inquiry about religion or creed be made. Any inquiries that indicate denomination or customs is unlawful. Applicants cannot be told that the organization is a Protestant, Catholic, or Jewish organization. Requesting a reference from a clergyman is also unlawful.

Birthplace/National Origin. Any attempt to inquire into the applicant's place of birth, the birthplace of relatives, or the national origin is unlawful, unless it is a BFOQ or job-related item.

Age. It is unlawful to discriminate against applicants in the forty to seventy age group under the Age Discrimination in Employment Act. EEOC decisions also make it unlawful to limit hiring to those within a predetermined age range. It is appropriate, however, to establish that the applicant is at least eighteen years of age. It is unlawful to require a birth certificate before hiring, but it may be requested after hiring. It is legal to request proof of age in the form of work permits issued by the school authorities.

Race/Color. Any inquiry related to race or color must be premised on the fact that the information is needed for job-related reasons. It is difficult to find an example of why race or color would be included in employment decision making, except for the EEO-1 job applicant log.

Height/Weight. Inquiry into height and weight is improper except in unusual situations wherein they are job-related.

Handicaps. It is proper to ask whether the applicant has any health problems—sensory, mental, or physical—that could affect job performance or job placement. General inquiries about handicaps that do not reasonably relate to an applicant's ability to perform a job would be considered unlawful; the courts are examining this area very carefully.

In *American National Insurance Company v. Fair Employment and Housing Commission*, 186 Cal. Rptr. 345, 651 P.2d 1151 (1982), the California Supreme Court held that an insurance company violated the California Fair Employment Practice Act by rejecting a life insurance debit agent for employment on the basis of his high blood pressure. The company believed employment would expose the agent to a greater than normal risk of disability or death even though it did not presently impair his ability to work. The court held that elevated blood pressure was protected as a physical handicap under the act, and the company's policy excluded persons with high blood pressure from employment regardless of ability to perform. The court stated that "the law clearly was designed to prevent employers from acting arbitrarily against physical conditions that, whether actually or potentially handicapping, may present no current job disability or job-related health risk."

In *Bentivegna v. U.S. Department of Labor,* 694 F.2d 619, 30 EPD ¶33,211 (CA-9, 1982), the U.S. Court of Appeals for the Ninth Circuit reinstated an employee with back pay to 1973 because he had been unlawfully discharged from the City of Los Angeles for uncontrolled diabetes. The handicapped employee was a construction carpenter. In this case, the city cited absenteeism, shortness of careers of diabetics with health problems, increased risk for infection, and prolonged healing time for minor injuries and infections. The court stated that when such "remote concerns ... legitimize discrimination" the intent of Section 504 of the Rehabilitation Act of 1973 is not operable. Even though many handicapped individuals have health problems that may affect attendance and work, these concerns are not an adequate basis for discriminatory job qualifications, except when they are related to "business necessity or safe performance on the job." For an example of this principle, *OFCCP v. Southern Pacific Transportation Co.,* 2 DLR 1983 A-2, and *Pacific Motor Trucking Company v. Bureau of Labor and Industries,* (Ore. Ct.App.) 192 DLR 1983 A-1, show that a back condition is a handicap.

One of the problems that these cases bring into focus concerns the question of the prospective employee's "medical condition" on the employment application. If the employee is rejected for high blood pressure, bad back, or diabetes and it cannot be shown that these conditions are "job-related," the person has been rejected for unlawful reasons. This could violate job handicap acts under both state and federal statutes applicable to the hospital involved.

Citizenship. The employer may ask the applicant whether he or she is a U.S. citizen. If not, the applicant may be asked if he or she intends to become one. Proof of citizenship may be required only after the individual is hired. The employer may not ask whether the applicant is native-born or naturalized and may not ask the applicant to answer these questions about his or her parents.

Photographs. An employer may require photographs after candidates have been hired when the photographs are utilized for identification purposes. They should not be required before hiring.

Education. It is lawful to inquire about the academic, professional, or vocational schools attended, as well as about reading, writing, and verbal ability in foreign languages. State licenses can be required in certain positions. It is unlawful to inquire about the nationality, racial, or religious nature of any educational institution, and it is imprudent to inquire about a language as a mother tongue or in relation to skill acquisition, unless such inquiries are job-related.

Because safety in the administration of medications is essential, many nurse orientation programs include a test on competency in mathematics. Institutions that adhere to this practice should take care to administer the test after hiring and to ensure that a valid, reliable instrument is used in optimal test conditions.

Relatives. It is proper to ask the name, relationship, and address of the individual who should be notified in case of emergency. Discriminatory questions about a relative are unlawful.

Organizations. It is lawful to ask about the organizations to which an applicant belongs, as long as such an inquiry excludes those based on union activity, handicap, race, color, religion, sex, national origin, or ancestry. The employer may ask what offices an applicant holds in such an organization.

Military Service. The employer may inquire about the applicant's tours of duty in the U.S. armed forces. The employer may also ask rank and branch of service and may require a military discharge certificate after the applicant has been hired. It is unlawful to request the military records or to ask about service in the military forces of countries other than the United States.

Work Schedule. It is appropriate and imperative to explain the work schedule that the applicant will have on the job for which the interview has been granted. The employer should inquire about the applicant's willingness to work said schedule.

Other Qualifications. Some jobs require special training or experience. Unusual questions must be justified in relation to their job-related nature.

Experience. It is lawful to ask about the applicant's work experience and about foreign countries to which the applicant has traveled.

Credit Rating. It is inadvisable to ask applicants about their credit rating, as it is difficult to support such an inquiry as job-related. This area of questioning raises concerns about the privacy of the individual. Many states have laws restricting what employers may obtain from private and public institutions in relation to credit history. Nearly a dozen states, however, have fair credit reporting laws that allow disclosure of credit ratings to an employer. Intercorporate sharing of data about individuals for use in evaluating prospective employees has sparked litigation. Much of the information that an employer gains from secondary sources can be gathered from applicants themselves if skillful interviewing techniques are used. The focal point in the interview is to determine what information is relevant to the job in question.

Criminal Record. Many employers wonder what they may ask in relation to the applicant's criminal record. Some states have laws restricting access to criminal or psychiatric history. Nineteen states prohibit or restrict the use of psychological stress tests or polygraph testing on potential employees.

It is not lawful to ask applicants about their arrest record, although it is appropriate to ask, "Have you ever been convicted of a crime other than traffic, game law, or other minor violations? If yes, give the nature of the offense and other circumstances regarding conviction." If the applicant has been convicted of a felony, the effect of such a conviction on employment status must be considered on a case by case basis. The EEOC has held that a minority applicant cannot be rejected for employment on the basis of a criminal record, *unless the criminal record is job-related.* For example, a convicted drug dealer should not work where there is access to drugs. A person convicted of auto theft, however, might be suited to a job as a cook in the cafeteria. Under Title VII of the Civil Rights Act of 1964, employment practices that are neutral in appearance, intent, and application become illegal when they operate to the disadvantage of a disproportionate number of minority applicants. Because more minority group members are convicted criminals, the employer must consider this issue carefully in selecting or rejecting certain individuals for this reason.

Marital Status/Family Status. Interviewers frequently ask applicants about children, ages of children, child care arrangements, and other general family-related matters as a means of showing interest in the applicants and helping them to relax. Such innocent questions can violate the rights of the applicants, however. More and more applicants are aware of their legal rights. Questions about the age and number of children or other dependents are also not appropriate. Asking a female applicant about how long she plans to remain employed or her future plans for pregnancy is not legal; such a conversation is discriminatory because the same questions would not be asked of a male applicant applying for the same post. It is appropriate to ask the applicant whether specific work schedules, commitments, activities, or responsibilities can be met. A good way to get the necessary information is to review the job description and the scheduling arrangement with the applicant during the interviewing process. Without asking direct questions, the interviewer might be able to use open-ended questions that encourage the applicant to talk freely.

Statement on Application. A notice may appear on the application to advise applicants that misstatements or omissions of material facts may result in dismissal. The following is an example of an appropriate statement:

> By completing and submitting this application I understand and agree that (1) any misstatement of material facts will be adequate cause for immediate withdrawal of this application or, in the event of employment, be deemed a cause for dismissal; (2) my previous employers and educational institutions may be asked for information concerning my employment, character, ability, and experience, and I release any person giving or receiving such information; (3) no question on this application has

been answered in such a way to disclose my race, color, religion, or national origin; (4) if employed, I will furnish proof of age by a birth certificate and any license that is required to perform my job; (5) I realize that my employment is terminable-at-will having no specific duration, and that this is not an employment contract and that I may be terminated by the hospital at any time without liability for wages or salary except that earned at the date of termination. I agree to search of my person or of any locker or property assigned to me, and hereby waive all claims for damages on account of such examination. I authorize any physician or hospital to release any information which may be necessary to determine my ability to perform the duties of a job I am being considered for prior to employment or in the future during my employment with the hospital; and (6) I understand that business needs make the following conditions: mandatory overtime, shift work, a rotating work schedule, or a work schedule other than Monday through Friday. I agree to these as conditions of my continuing employment and that the hospital may change wages, benefits, and conditions at any time.

This disclaimer should appear on the employment application form rather than an employee handbook, because the latter often falls into the hands of union organizers. An enterprising union organizer would not have the terminable-at-will statement in item 5 since he or she would not see the employment application. Further, it is unwise to ever expressly state in an employee handbook that an employee can be terminated *without cause*. It would be difficult for the hospital to ever meet the campaign propaganda that it reserves the right to discharge employees without cause.

Selection of Employees

Before they can pick optimal employees, managers must examine hospital and departmental philosophy, purpose, and objectives; then they must relate these general criteria to specific, objective, performance-based criteria that are part of a behaviorally stated job description. When the job criteria have been formulated, the same standards must be used in the evaluation of each applicant. Qualifications, physical limits related to criteria spelled out for the job, and references should always be verified. References suggested by the applicant tend to focus on positive comments, regardless of the total circumstances. Positive references should be taken with a grain of salt. Questionable references always should be pursued, particularly with the applicant.

Before the interview begins, the interviewer should review hospital policies and procedures, as well as the job description of the position for which a qualified candidate is sought, and should formulate job-related questions. The interviewer may recap a recent problem and ask the applicant for an opinion on problem management; for example, "We at XYZ hospital have just implemented the primary nursing care concept. We find some intershift conflict. Tell me about your experience with primary nursing care. What do you suggest to improve team building between the shifts?" The following interview techniques should be helpful:

KEY POINTS:

...The interviewer should listen more than half of the time.

...Adequate data and validation of facts are essential in formulating conclusions.

...Avoid leading the applicant toward desired responses.

...Reflect on the points that the employee or prospective employee emphasized.

In an actual interview, you would also be able to assess your comprehensiveness and effectiveness by learning about how much information you gleaned on the following:

1. Academic skills and aptitudes
   A. Thought patterns/organization
   B. Communication skills
   C. General resource organization and utilization
   D. Personal and nursing philosophies
   E. Analytic ability
   F. General knowledge

2. Motivation
   A. Goals
   B. Ability to follow through
   C. Interests/significant motivating factors
   D. Professional commitment
   E. Real versus ideal expectations

3. Personality
   A. Body language
   B. Self-concept and direction
   C. Strengths
   D. Ability to get along with others

4. Experience
   A. Insight

   B. Efforts at remaining current
   C. Leadership, attempts to research issues, apply knowledge, and innovate as appropriate
   D. Experience at other jobs
5. Job suitability
   A. Agreement with hospital mission and goals
   B. Acceptance of policies and procedures
   C. Understanding of/agreement with job role and functions[1]

Conversation can be facilitated if the interviewer takes the following steps:

1. Structure items for which specific information is required.
2. Formulate some open-ended questions.
3. Utilize direct eye contact.
4. Arrange your seating arrangement to optimize power or informality, as you desire.
5. Do not make promises to the employee if you are uncertain about their getting the job. Don't promise a job for a specific duration.
6. Use questions such as the following ones to gain insight into the interviewee's assessment and thinking processes:
   - What do you expect from us? How can we meet your needs?
   - What will your last supervisor tell me are your two strongest/weakest points?
   - How does this job relate to your future plans?
   - If you were hiring someone for this job, what qualities would you look for?
   - Why do you have that particular goal, problem, or situation?
   - What makes you tick?
   - Are you more comfortable following or leading?...Why?
7. It is also useful and helpful to ask the interviewees about why they seek employment at your agency/hospital, and what they know about you. Interviewees who have done some research on your agency deserve an A for effort.[2]
8. Find out the circumstances concerning the applicants' leaving their previous jobs, what they enjoyed best and least of the previous jobs, and what they feel are their greatest strengths.

When documenting the progress of an employment interview, the interviewer should limit the comments written on the applicant's file to job-related statements.

No psychological interpretation of behavior and statements, such as "She was pushy." or "He was militant." should be noted; only the facts of the applicant's responses to criteria stipulated in the policies, procedures, and job description should be included in the file.

Tone of Orientation

Employers should attempt to delineate disciplinary standards and the hospital's major philosophies from their first contact with an employee. Every attempt should be made to show employees that standards are equitably and consistently applied. Orientation is a good time to initiate this practice.

Checklists can be used to ensure that the performance of each employee in a given category is evaluated according to the same standard. Published policies and procedures, which may comprise an implied contract between the employer and the employee should be emphasized. The permissible orientation period and probation should be determined by the hospital's probationary policy and the new employee's job ability.

New nurses may suffer from so-called bicultural adaptation because the reality of the work deviates significantly from what school represented as reality. The adjustment and the skills acquisition period may take up to one year for a new graduate. This adjustment period is not only very stressful for the new graduate but also expensive for the hospital. Marlene Kramer has a program designed to facilitate the transition for new graduates.[3,4]

Hospitals with institutionwide education departments must work hard to ensure that good starts in orientation do not fall by the wayside when the new employee goes to the work area. Moreover, if the education department does not receive the necessary feedback, the orientation period may not be used to maximal advantage. Continuity by the education department as well as other appropriate departments receiving feedback on the new employees is important. In too many hospitals, this continuity is lost because of power struggles and territorial claims by various department managers.

PERFORMANCE APPRAISALS

In any discrimination complaint, performance appraisals are generally scrutinized carefully because most employment decisions—layoffs, promotions, merit raises, discharges, transfers, or special training requests—are based on these evaluations. The performance appraisal can be defined as a periodic, formal evaluation of job performance over a specified time frame. Too often, supervisors rate an employee's performance average as good simply because they do not want to confront the employee. These appraisals may cause problems in later discrimination cases, however.

These evaluations are used to

1. determine job competency
2. motivate personnel toward higher objectives
3. identify staff development needs generally and specifically
4. learn about employee talents, strengths, aspirations, and weaknesses
5. improve communication between management and the staff
6. clarify expectations on role behaviors and job performance
7. examine strategies for improving job performance
8. reward commendable job efforts
9. select employees for promotion, layoff, transfer, raises, or special training
10. identify unsatisfactory performance so that corrective action can be taken[5-9]

Correlation with Job Description

The traditional job description is deficient in two ways. It fails to identify the complete performance expected of an employee, and it does not explain the relationship between those standards that are listed and what skills and minimum qualifications are needed for the expected performance. Traditionally, managers have assumed that the job description is a vague summary of a job, whereas the performance appraisal relates to the behaviors of the employee in the job. These documents have been input-oriented and, thus, have failed to deal with quantity, quality, or timeliness of a service or with standards that vary with changing conditions. It is time to stop basing performance appraisals for individuals on a standard, too often weakly defined, that is separate from the job description.

Output-oriented job descriptions, on the other hand, lend themselves to recruitment, goal setting, and standard setting for performance appraisals. Such appraisals can be used as an objective means of assessing group and individual employee performance in relation to budgetary planning, productivity, and other parameters of performance important to a hospital. An output-oriented job description ensures that hiring, orientation, and daily work practices are developed around a common standard. This eliminates the problem of discrepancies between what employees believe a given job comprises and what managers want. The new type of job description should retain a specific job title, a code that can be used in leveling and classifying the job, a statement of accountability and reporting responsibilities, and the hazards—biopsychosocial, environmental, and chemical—inherent in the work.

To state jobs in terms of output, it is necessary to break the job description down into modules wherein for each task the conditions of performance, the standards of acceptable minimum compliance, skills, knowledge, abilities, and qualifications are delineated (Exhibit 9–1). This method has a number of advantages and disadvantages, and no one has the perfect format for developing such a job description. The format of output-oriented job descriptions is a task for the 1980s. The advantages of this type of job description include:

- ability to relate organizational inputs to outputs
- tool to assist managers in orienting new employees to performance expectations
- provision of data necessary for the organization as a whole to establish objectives
- criteria provided for use in making performance appraisals
- feedback mechanism to let employees know the standards for promotions
- well-delineated concept of what employees do in terms that promote communication among the entire hospital management team

One disadvantage is that a job description specific to each position in the hospital must be written; furthermore, it must be rewritten when conditions or standards change. In patient care areas, however, the data retrieved from computerized patient classification systems can simplify this process. For example, a nurse who is expected to care for eight patients at a certain level of care when the acuity is at level II, can be expected to provide total care for only six seriously ill

---

Exhibit 9–1 Output-Oriented Job Description

Module	Components Specified
Tasks	Behaviors, duties, or functions that are important to the employee's job.
Conditions	How often is a given task done?
	What conditions hinder or facilitate the performance of the task?
	What policies, procedures, directions, or educational resources are available to assist the employee in task completion?
	What other departments or resource people should the employee consult for assistance?
Requirements	Skills, knowledge, abilities, and experiences required to perform task; exceptions to these requirements for times of short staffing.
	(*Note:* Evaluate this item in relation to comparable worth concept.)
Qualifications	What education, special training, or experience is needed to ensure that employees have the requisite skills, knowledge, abilities, and experience to perform the task?

patients when the acuity is at level III. For example, an actual census of twenty may be an effective census of twenty-seven or more. (An *effective* census is calculated on the basis of patient needs and acuity; it may differ from the *actual* census in numbers of patients.)

As employees move into higher level positions, it is more difficult to specify the exact tasks that they perform. Typical tasks may be included in the job description as examples. Items of responsibility can be handled by permitting executives to write a contract on what they can be expected to perform in a given time period. Such a contract can be written using an objectives format that identifies deadlines and specific outcomes.

To keep people from saying "That is not in my job description" as an excuse to avoid certain tasks, a general catchall phrase that makes the employee responsible for all other assigned duties should be included. Moreover, if typical examples of expectations are included, they should be accompanied by a statement that the descriptors specified are not exclusive and job performance will not be confined to these descriptors.

Not all labor relations experts believe that management should have actual job descriptions. The majority of the staff, professionals included, will want very specific job descriptions, i.e., job ownership. An enlightened manager, however, will want job flexibility. In a health care setting where accountability is assigned and various legal implications must be considered, a job description should be results-oriented, but should allow flexibility for group participation if possible.

GOALS OF THE PERFORMANCE APPRAISAL

The outcome-based job description becomes a valuable tool for the supervisor who must rate the individual employee on actual job performance. Many health care leaders are also advocating some space on the performance appraisal in which the employee and manager may together identify areas for goal setting. For example, they may set a goal to:

improve communications and services for clients by:

- writing a care plan on all assigned new admissions
- adding to and updating care plans on assigned patients
- spending time with patients who have great emotional needs
- explaining the procedure and rationale to patients who are undergoing diagnostic testing
- making referrals to other departments, e.g., social worker, chaplain, or public health department, as appropriate

This objective will be evaluated daily by the head nurse. Acceptable performance will be determined by documented evidence on the nursing notes and care plan and by interviews with patients. Feedback to the employee will be continual. A formal summary of progress in improving practice with patients will be made on April 15, 19XX after the employee has attended two training sessions on patient communications and care plan writing, scheduled for Jan. 19th and Feb. 7th, and has had time to change work habits.

The objective setting component of the performance appraisal tool can be utilized to motivate a good employee in attaining higher goals. This tool is also invaluable in creating and maintaining healthy upward and downward communications.

Bias-Free Performance Appraisals

In order to avoid later discrimination charges, a performance appraisal should be written to include both the good and the bad of an employee's performance. This provides factual support for any later decisions involving the employee. The following suggestions can be helpful in documenting a case:

1. Managers should be familiar with the exact performance level that the employee exhibits prior to the appraisal meeting.
2. Boxes or items on the performance appraisal should not be checked if they do not apply to the employee. For example, "Supervises others well" is not applicable to a beginning typist who does not supervise anyone.
3. Comments describing employee behaviors should be very specific. "Lacks motivation" is insufficient. The manager should say that "Ms. X never offers to assist other team members when her work assignment is completed before theirs is done."
4. Comments on employee appearance, values, or personal attitudes should be avoided unless these can be directly related to the job performance.
5. The manager should take time to review the evaluation with another manager to be certain that ratings are objective and justifiable in relation to job expectations required of all employees in the same classification.
6. None of the information should come as a surprise to the employee. Effective managers give employees constant feedback on their expectations and employee performance. The performance appraisal is merely a formal document that summarizes this performance at specified intervals.

Rewarding the Managers

Organizations are always giving managers priorities. Too often, managers, who work hard to comply with requests, feel that they are never equitably rewarded.

Every organization should consider whether its managers are appropriately rewarded when they go the extra mile to develop employees. Do managers have the necessary training to (1) document the performance appraisal process in a legally defensible and practical way; (2) share the appraisal process with their employees; (3) know the goals and direction of the organization well enough to interpret it to employees; (4) approach the session as a problem-solving, counseling session, instead of only as an administrative act; and (5) utilize information from these evaluations to create programs that will positively affect the staff? If managers work hard to obtain the extra training and implement a progressive program of development, are they rewarded? If not, the organization may find that managers lack the enthusiasm to make evaluations more than an administrative procedure and their failure to communicate positive feelings to their employees may create a morale problem.

ADMINISTRATION OF DISCIPLINE[10]

Discipline is a major factor in keeping employees happy and in remaining a union-free employer. There are no pat formulas, however. What works well in one situation may not work at other times. No matter how they handle the situation, the managers' goals should be to make the employee appropriately responsible, to recognize and acknowledge positive behaviors and performance, to reinforce the employee's personal sense of worth, and to make the employee feel like an important member of the team. Managers must remember that unions look for:

- unhappy workers who need deserved recognition
- workers who are overqualified for jobs
- workers with unsatisfactory performance and inappropriate behavior
- supervisors who play favorites
- complainers who have not been heard
- workers who "get away with" poor performance
- inconsistent disciplinary policies

A favorite target of union organizers is management's absolute control of discipline and discharge.

Discipline can be defined as the process of correcting, educating, and directing employees to comply with reasonable, practical rules that pertain to behavioral expectations and constraints. A firm policy on discipline should be adopted and publicized as follows:

It is basic to our personnel relations policy that the purpose of disciplinary action is to correct the offender's shortcomings, rather than to punish. An employee will be discharged only when other discipline is deemed inappropriate by management. Any employee who requires corrective action will be appropriately warned, unless the offense is sufficiently serious to merit discharge without a specific prior warning.

Rule enforcement must be consistent across and among the affected group. An appeals procedure should be available for discharge cases. Reasons for disciplinary action include:

- chronic absenteeism
- unreported absence
- tardiness
- drinking or use of drugs on duty
- insubordination
- dishonesty
- garnishments
- failure to follow instructions, procedures
- fighting on organizational premises
- leaving without permission
- housekeeping duties, e.g., keeping your work area neat
- improper conduct, swearing
- reporting to work under the influence of alcohol or drugs or possessing these substances on duty
- violation of safety rules
- carelessness
- destruction of organizational property
- defective and improper work
- theft
- no distribution/no solicitation (must be carefully stated, particularly in regard to "actual working time")
- falsifying information on the employment application, leave of absence forms, time records, medical records, financial records or any other official records of the hospital
- absence from work for three days without having given proper notice
- gambling on hospital property
- recording time on another employee's time card or letting another employee do the same for you
- unauthorized possession of weapon on duty

- divulging confidential information about patients or their families
- physical or verbal abuse of a patient
- sleeping on duty
- any conduct viewed to be in active disregard of hospital or patient interest

Disciplinary policies should include a statement at the end, similar to the following: "The commission of these infractions will result in disciplinary action up to and including discharge, depending on the seriousness of the offense in the judgment of management." The examples given are not an exhaustive list of all possible behavioral or performance deficiencies that could result in disciplinary action. Each department head is responsible and authorized to define additional reasonable performance standards appropriate to their respective areas.

Many supervisors dread, and even postpone, the one-to-one meeting in which they must discipline an employee. No one wants to bear bad news. For these reasons, many disciplinary sessions are done incorrectly and/or may be delayed long beyond the time when they should occur.

Know the Facts

Before managers administer discipline, they must:

1. state and document organizational rules and consequences of failure to comply with specific policies and procedures
2. get specific details on:

- employee work history;
- interim behavioral and performance appraisals;
- past problems, measures taken, and employee responses; and
- current behavioral and/or performance problems

3. be sure that facts are dated, verified, objective, and complete
4. seek input from appropriate co-workers, managers, clients, and others
5. allow the employee to fully state his or her side of the story before reaching any final conclusions
6. be prepared to defend their action to legal representatives, superiors, and the board of directors
7. document ways that they have provided skills, time, knowledge, or supervised practice to qualify the employee to meet requirements and expectations
8. determine if this matter requires progressive discipline or immediate suspension or discharge.

At this point, managers should ask themselves:

- How have I handled similar cases in the past?
- How do other department heads handle this type of problem?
- Am I discriminating against this individual?
- Have personality conflicts clouded my decision?
- Does the corrective action fit the violation?
- How will my actions avoid a recurrence of this problem for this employee and others?
- What kind of impact will my decision have on morale?
- Will my approach to discipline inspire this employee to improve his or her behavior and performance?
- Have I checked this decision with my supervisor or management peer?
- Should I take corrective action on this employee or on the group collectively?
- Can I explain my actions to the employee?
- Can I explain the significance of this problem to the employee in understandable terms?
- Do I have specific ideas on how this employee can avoid this problem in the future?
- Am I ready to handle any resentment that the employee might express?

Interview the Employee

The following suggestions can assist managers in the disciplinary interview:

1. Come to the meeting with written notes on the specific details of the situation, organizational policy relating to these behaviors, prior corrective remedies, standard on-the-job training, and orientation materials relating to the problem at hand. Have a written plan of corrective actions that are appropriate to the situation and include a range of possibilities.
2. Arrange the meeting as a private session in which only those directly involved in the action or the discipline are in attendance.
3. Provide adequate time for a complete discussion of the problem and any corrective remedies.
4. Set a serious tone for the meeting. Review your understanding of the problem with the employee. Allow the employee to explain his or her perception of the problem.
5. After both you and the employee have presented the facts, explain:

- the seriousness of the situation
- the corrective action
- criteria for acceptable performance
- deadlines for improvement
- the meaning of this event to this employee and to other employees
- this employee's future in the organization

6. Do not violate the employee's Weingarten rights as explained later in this chapter.

Suggest specific measures, training, or behavioral changes that the employee may utilize in complying with the stated expectations. If the employee is upset or if the business is unfinished, offer to continue the discussion at an appropriate other date and time.

It is reasonable to expect employees to be accountable for all policies, rules, and procedures, as well as to make a conscientious effort to correct established performance deficiencies. Consultation with the personnel director is advisable when corrective action is needed to ensure that the manager directing the employee meeting complies with legal requirements and hospital procedures.

Take Corrective Action

Unless the case is extreme, the employee should have an oral warning before receiving an official, documented warning. Organizational standards should be set for various offenses, since it is critical that corrective action taken for similar offenses be consistent throughout the hospital. An oral warning should be dated and placed in the employee file. All events leading to more than an oral warning, such as a formal reprimand, should be thoroughly documented by the involved manager on the day that the incident occurred and the documentation placed in the employee file.

No manager should have the power to fire a person on the spot. At most, the employee should be suspended until a complete investigation of the facts can be made. All statements of others relating to the investigation should be written as part of the record. It is also *very* important to have all admissions written verbatim. That which the employee claims as support of his or her position should also be a part of the record. Unless the offense is serious enough for discharge, the first offense normally results in an oral warning. The second offense ends in a written warning; the third, a disciplinary layoff; the fourth, discharge.

Documenting the Disciplinary Action

It is wise to devise a policy or a file form that shows the specific components of any disciplinary process. Categories that may be included are:

- significant data, e.g., name, date, job title, type of employment, length of employment
- problem
- supporting facts and anecdotal incidents
- organizational policy relating to this problem
- standard on-the-job training or orientation that relates to this issue
- corrective action taken
- criteria and deadlines for evaluating employee response to corrective action
- specific training, counseling, follow-up indicated for this problem
- date for next conference or exit interview for those who have been terminated
- final outcome and evaluation
- supporting facts and anecdotal incidents relating to final decision and action
- some form of dated written notice to the employee that has been signed by the employee and supervisor; a mechanism for employee and supervisor comments

SAMPLE PROBLEMS IN DISCIPLINARY SITUATIONS

Before implementing disciplinary measures, managers must ensure that their corrective actions do not violate the law. There are a number of ways that such violations can occur.

Violation of the Occupational Safety and Health Act

The Occupational Safety and Health Act of 1970 (29 U.S.C.S. Section 651, et. seq.) provides the Secretary of Labor authority to promulgate mandatory federal health standards applicable to every private employer in a business affecting commerce. The law includes a "general duty" clause under which employers are required to maintain work places free from "recognized hazards" that are causing, or are likely to cause, death or serious bodily harm. The Department of Labor, through its secretary, is charged with the duty to see that the act is complied with and charges by any employee that the employer is not in compliance may be made to the department through the regional office. Also, the Department of Labor's Occupational Safety and Health Administration (OSHA) inspectors initiate their own inspections through a priority system. If, upon inspection or investigation, the inspector believes an employer is guilty of violating the act, he will issue a citation to the employer. This citation can be appealed to the Occupational Safety and Health Review Commission, made up of three members appointed by the President for six-year terms. The commission operates and has the same investigatory powers as those given the NLRB under the Labor Management Relations Act, 1947, as amended.

Under OSHA, the Secretary of Labor passed a federal regulation (29 CFR § 1977.12(b)(2)) that provides under Section 11(c)(1) of the act that an employer is prohibited from discharging or discriminating against any employee who exercises his right to not perform a task due to a reasonable apprehension of death or serious injury coupled with a reasonable belief that no alternative is available. This federal regulation came under scrutiny in the case of *Whirlpool Corporation v. Marshall*, 100 S.Ct. 883, 445 U.S. 1 (1980), described as follows:

> At its plant in Marion, Ohio, overhead conveyors transport appliance components throughout the plant. To protect employees from objects that occasionally fall from these conveyors, Whirlpool had installed a horizontal wire-mesh guard screen approximately twenty feet above the plant floor. This mesh screen was welded to angle-iron frames suspended from the building's structural steel skeleton.
>
> Maintenance employees of Whirlpool spend several hours each week removing objects from the screen, replacing paper spread on the screen to catch grease drippings from the material on the conveyors and performing occasional maintenance work on the conveyors themselves. To perform these duties, maintenance employees usually are able to stand on the iron frames, but sometimes find it necessary to step onto the steel mesh screen itself.
>
> In 1973, Whirlpool had begun to install heavier wire in the screen because its safety had been questioned. Several employees had fallen partly through the old screen and on one occasion, an employee had fallen completely through to the plant floor below but had survived.
>
> Then, in 1974, a maintenance employee fell to his death through the guard screen where the newer, stronger mesh had not been installed. Two maintenance men voiced complaints a few weeks later.
>
> The next day, the two employees reported for the night shift. Their foreman walked on some of the angle-iron frames and directed the two men to perform their usual maintenance duties on a section of the old screen. The maintenance men claimed that the screen was unsafe and refused to carry out this directive. The foreman then sent them to the personnel office. They were ordered to punch out without working or being paid for the remaining six hours of the shift. The two subsequently received written reprimands that were placed in their employment files.

In the *Whirlpool* case, although OSHA does not require employers to pay workers who refuse a task in the face of imminent danger, it does provide that employers may not discriminate against workers for such refusals by placing written reprimands in their files.

Whirlpool argued that to allow the employees to refuse to do a job would give workers the power to shut down a work site—a power denied by Congress even to OSHA inspectors, because it would give unilateral authority to federal officials without judicial safeguards.

The U.S. District Court for the Southern District of Ohio ruled that the regulation promulgated by the Secretary of Labor pursuant to the Occupational Safety and Health Act was invalid. The Court of Appeals, Sixth Circuit, at 593 F.2d 715, reversed and Whirlpool appealed this decision to the Supreme Court. The Supreme Court held that there was no right afforded by OSHA that would entitle employees to walk off the job because of potential unsafe conditions at the workplace.

However, circumstances may sometimes exist in which the employee justifiably believes that the express statutory arrangement does not sufficiently protect him or her from death or serious injury if the job is completed.

The Supreme Court found that the regulation (29 C.F.R. § 1977.12 (b) (c)) was a valid exercise of the Labor Department's authority under OSHA and constituted a permissible interpretation of the act in light of its language, structure, and legislative history.

The key questions to ask in cases involving refusal of a direct order due to a good faith belief that the job presents imminent danger are: "Has this job been done by this employee or others without any accidents occurring?" "Have the employees been given the proper safety training from an experienced safety official to show how the job can be performed correctly?" "Is this the kind of job that does, in fact, pose imminent danger to life or limb?"

Protected Concerted Activity

In *Ontario Knife Co.*, 247 NLRB 168 (1980), a non-union company employed some three hundred employees on both day and night shifts. Employee Cobado worked with two other night shift employees, Biggs and Swift. Among other things, they riveted handles to machetes. Cobado and Swift had complained for a long time over what they considered to be an excessive assignment of machete work to the night shift. Both Cobado and Swift told night shift foreman Peterson that, the next time it was their turn to work on machetes, they were going to refuse. The foreman cussed and replied that they were to do whatever work he assigned them. At this, Cobado packed up her belongings and walked off the job. The next day she telephoned the personnel manager to tell him her side of the story and to ask if she were still eligible to come to work. She was told that she had been terminated for walking off the job and the plant manager took responsibility for that decision.

Employee Cobado filed unfair labor practice charges with the National Labor Relations Board (NLRB), claiming that the company violated the NLRA by firing her for engaging in protected concerted activities, in that she and her fellow employees had complained of the alleged unfair distribution of machete work on the night shift. While the result of this case is somewhat circuitous, it is important, since parallel situations could happen in nursing staffs on the night shift who may complain they receive all the hard work and then possibly walk off the job if their complaint is not answered.

In *Ontario Knife Company*, the NLRB said:

> The Administrative Law Judge (ALJ) found, and we agree, that the machete grievance discussion was protected concerted activity. The ALJ further found that, if Swift had walked out with Cobado in protest of the above, the walkout also would have been protected concerted activity. He (ALJ) concluded, however that Cobado's walkout was a personal decision resulting from Peterson's remarks and was therefore unprotected. He (ALJ) found Cobado's discharge for leaving the plant without permission was not a violation of 8(a)(1) of the Act, and he dismissed the Complaint.

The NLRB disagreed with their Administrative Law Judge's finding that Cobado's walkout was unprotected and not a violation of the NLRA. It stated:

> Even assuming, arguendo, that Peterson's statement about kissing his *** caused Cobado's walkout, the statements must be considered in the context of the entire conversation, which was clearly protected concerted activity...Indeed, Peterson's remarks conveyed the message that Peterson *was unwilling to consider seriously* the machete complaint. When this was made clear to Cobado, she walked out in protest. It is well-settled that employees have the right to leave work in support of a grievance pertaining to terms and conditions of employment. When this occurs, an Employer may not lawfully discipline an employee for breaking a Company rule concerning leaving work without permission; for to allow it would abrogate the statutory right to withhold services in support of a grievance (Emphasis supplied).

However, on appeal, the court overruled this decision.

Two points are pertinent in applying the principles of this case. First, employees at a non-union company can leave work without permission if they do it *concertedly,* and if their complaint relates to legitimate concerns over wages or conditions of employment. For example, if employees leave work to protest it being too cold, an employer cannot fire them; however, the employer can permanently replace them. If Cobado's employer had hired a new permanent replacement during the day she left, the employer would not have to fire her and she still would have been permanently replaced.

Second, if there had been a union on the scene with a collective bargaining agreement, including a typical no-strike clause and a grievance and arbitration procedure, employee Cobado would have violated the contract when she left work without permission, as she would have violated the well-established rule of "work now and grieve later." In this case, a union-represented employee could have fewer rights.

Weingarten Rights

The extent of an employee's right to counsel during a disciplinary or investigative interview is important in the health care industry, because the issue arises in many common situations and supervisors and employees do not always understand their rights and responsibilities.

In the case of *Ball Plastics,* 257 NLRB No. 126 (1981), a union had just been voted in and a first labor contract had been negotiated. Approximately one week later, a female employee who had worked for the company for sixteen years was discharged for refusing to do a job she did not think was in her job description. She felt that she was being treated unfairly because there were girls with less seniority than herself doing easier work. When she complained to her supervisor, he instructed her to return to the job. She refused and told him that she wanted to see her union steward. Her supervisor denied this request and told her to go back on her job. She refused.

The progression of events so far maintains the company's legal position. However, instead of suspending her for not doing her assigned job, her supervisor went to his general supervisor, who also asked her to go back to work. She again refused, and the general supervisor took her to the personnel manager, who again interviewed her about the work refusal. She did not ask the general supervisor or the personnel manager for a union steward, but she continued to refuse to do her assigned work. She was then taken to the plant manager, who did not grant her request to assign her to the foiling job, that she felt was a job in her job classification; the plant manager told her to return to the job she had refused to do. Again, she asked to see the union steward. The plant manager told her to return to work and contact the union steward on her own time. She refused. She was then sent back to personnel and terminated for insubordination. In the ensuing case, the Administrative Law Judge and the Board held that

> Under §7 of the Act, the employee has a right to union representation, or
> to another employee to represent her or him, at an investigatory inter-

view which the employee *reasonably believes* might result in disciplinary action. *NLRB v. J. Weingarten, Inc.*, 420 U.S. 251 (1975).

The supervisor should have suspended the employee and done nothing further with the employee until after the request for a union steward had been satisfied.

Managers should know that, even if a union does not yet represent employees, but is only organizing them, an employee has a right to have a union representative present if an interview is being conducted to investigate facts that could lead to an employee's discharge or discipline. (See *ITT Lighting Fixtures v. NLRB*, [CA-6, 1983] 200 DLR 1983: A-3.) The employee must request such representation, however. The best thing to do when an employee requests a union representative at a meeting is to terminate the meeting and seek appropriate legal advice.

Summary of Key Learning Principles

If an employee wants to have some other employee or a union representative for assistance while he or she is being interviewed by a supervisor or "higher-up" concerning a matter that could result in disciplinary action, do the following:

1. Bring the requested employee or union representative or end the interview.
2. Always bring in the higher-up managers upon employee request.
3. Watch out for *protected concerted activity* and employees complaining in groups.

The important point is that when you have the power to discharge at will, it is important to "walk the extra mile" with the employee and follow exact company procedures. If everything possible has been done and there still is a chronic complainer or malingerer, that individual must be warned according to policy and terminate him or her.

No matter how emotional a corrective action situation becomes, avoid swearing, threats, or inappropriate comments.

Watch for safety complaints. (See chapter 10 for types of complaints prevalent in hospitals.)

In summary, managers should remember that it is not the act of complaining, engaging in protected concerted activity, or complaining over safety and health hazards that they are disciplining them for, it is the employees' refusal to do their job because of groundless complaints, wherein genuine fear of imminent danger is lacking. Be sure that there is no imminent danger by checking the equipment or process in question. Also be sure that the employee has followed the work now, grieve later rule in the labor agreement or the complaint procedure in a union-free hospital.

The Troubled Employee

While intrinsic and extrinsic rewards are helpful in motivating the worker who is basically healthy, but failing to perform for a temporary period, they may not be sufficient to motivate the troubled employee. In addition to readily apparent physical problems, some employees have problems related to drug use, alcohol abuse, and psychological disturbances.

There are about ten million alcoholic workers in the U.S. work force today. In addition to the nearly $12.5 billion lost in productivity, these alcoholics are absent and involved in work-related accidents more often than are non-alcoholics. The high stress, sagging economy, inflation, high unemployment, and failing marriages of the 1980s also affect many hospital workers. Such problems cause emotional havoc that is frequently brought into the work place. Troubled employees are poorly motivated; turn out a poor work product; make excessive errors; are absent or tardy more often than others; waste time, energy, and resources; and have accidents or incidents of error more commonly than do others.

A number of solutions are available to managers who must deal with the troubled employee. For example, the manager may follow the disciplinary policy to the point of properly discharging the employee. Sometimes, managers do not want to fire the troubled employee and solve the problem by finding an out-of-the-way job for the employee that minimizes responsibility and contact or by transferring the employee to another department. The compromise solutions are actually unwise and costly, however, since they decrease the employee's self-esteem while forcing the hospital to create a bad precedent and absorb labor costs with diminishing returns. Condoning such conduct prohibits not only the subsequent discharge of this employee, but also that of other employees for similar conduct.

One large corporation pioneered an approach that can be of benefit in hospitals. Supervisors are trained to spot telltale signs of psychosocial problems in an employee. They then work to help the employee admit the problem and seek appropriate professional treatment. Any treatment that the employee receives is confidential and does not become part of the personnel file. The company records only that the employee is continuing in the appropriate program. When the treatment is complete, the employee returns to the work environment. Further treatment needs or corrective action is determined by the response of the employee, the opinion of the medical consultant, and the supervisor. This program has a positive psychological effect on employees who worry that they may be temporarily dysfunctional because of circumstances beyond their control. It is important in this type of program to monitor carefully those who are using it in order to take advantage of the system. Of course, if the employee fails to accept the problem or improve performance, termination is a frequent outcome.

ABSENTEEISM

The topic of absenteeism is frequently raised in managerial circles.[11] Because it adversely affects both morale and productivity, many different formulas and policies are being used to discipline employees for absenteeism. Incentive programs of all types are also commonly tried. Different programs are successful with different employees and hospitals, but there is a standard approach that should be part of any program.

The most effective way to control absenteeism is through supervisory contact, counseling, and follow-up with employees. To implement this approach, managers should be trained in ways to confront employees in a positive, constructive manner. Such an approach is predicated on the problem-solving method. Their immediate supervisor should talk to all employees who have been absent within one day of their return. At this talk, the supervisor asks each employee in a sincere way about the problem that caused the work absence. If the absence follows a pattern, the employee is reminded of that and warned about future implications of such behavior. If the employee has a problem or has been truly ill, the supervisor helps obtain further assistance or may modify the work schedule to allow the employee to resolve the problem. The purpose of the confrontation is not to force sick employees to return to work before they should, but to make system abusers think twice before they take advantage of the system. This method also lets employees know that management is aware of their personal needs. With this method, corrective counseling and assistance with problems can begin at the grass roots level.

Employees will not view this approach as an invasion of their privacy if managers show the same genuine concern across the board. For example, everyone seems to dislike floating to another work area. This duty is made more pleasant if the manager makes a point of thanking employees personally for working in an area other than their primary duty area when necessary. This approach falls nicely into the new management theories that emphasize the people skills. Employees with good attendance records appreciate the fact that the 20 percent of the people who take 80 percent of the time off are monitored and prevented from abusing the system. The result is better morale and increased productivity.

NOTES

1. Barbara Lang Rutkowski, *Nursing Leadership: Challenges and Dilemmas* (Evansville, IN: Nurse Consultation Services, 1981), pp. 64, 65.

2. Ibid., p. 66.

3. Marlene Kramer, *Reality Shock: Why Nurses Leave Nursing* (St. Louis: C. V. Mosby, 1974).

4. Carol S. Weisman et al., "Employment Patterns among Newly Hired Hospital Staff Nurses," *Nursing Research* 30 (May-June 1981): 180–191.

5. Thomas Alewine, "Performance Appraisals and Performance Standards," *Personnel Journal* 61 (March 1982): 210–213.

6. Arthur Brief, "Developing a Usable Performance Appraisal System," *Journal of Nursing Administration* 9 (October 1979): 7–10.

7. Jon D. Council and Roger J. Plachy, "Performance Appraisal Is Not Enough," *Journal of Nursing Administration* (October 1980): 20–26.

8. Bruce McAfee, "Performance Appraisal: Whose Function?" *Personnel Journal* 60 (April 1981): 298–299.

9. Rosa-Fay Milnar, "Performance Analysis—A How To," *Supervisor Nurse* 12 (February 1981): 14–15.

10. The material in this section is adapted from Arthur D. Rutkowski, *Working Together* (Evansville, IN: Nurse Consultation Services, 1981).

11. J. Michael McDonald, "What Is Your Absenteeism IQ?" *Personnel Journal* 59 (May-June 1980): 33–37.

Chapter 10

Legal Trends and
Supportable Positions

In today's litigious society, it is becoming much more difficult to defend a discharge decision. Common litigation in the 1980s are wrongful discharge suits filed by disgruntled former employees based on race, sex, or age discrimination; torts of outrageous discharge; negligent terminations; or allegations that the discharge is a breach of an implied contract created by an employee handbook.

EQUAL OPPORTUNITY EMPLOYMENT

Because hospitals employ members of many minority groups, they are particularly vulnerable to certain legal actions and to unionization. A study of various union strategies used in organizing nurses, for example, indicates that part of a union's appeal is its promise to correct discriminatory practices, advance women's rights, and promote the concept of comparable worth. A union may seem to be a viable option to nurses because it offers them an alternative remedy to their problems and a readily available, empathetic support system.

Enlightened administrators are working rapidly to remove discrimination from organizational practice. Equitable treatment of employees is increasingly demanded by contemporary employees. Managers can utilize their efforts to provide equal opportunities as a way to enhance employees' good feelings about working in a given setting. Such efforts are also important for managers to use in an organizing attempt. Managers not only must advocate equity in employment practices, however, but also must defend themselves against employees who file charges and lawsuits in personnel decisions that are not to their liking. The legal requirements for developing defensible personnel decisions are vague, ambiguous, and constantly changing because of new court decisions and societal trends. Even so, it is imperative that management develop some practical ways of defending personnel decisions and practices.

In the health care industry, men, women, and members of minorities are found to have fairly predictable jobs. Most of the cases handled by the Equal Employment Opportunity Commission (EEOC) seem to be concerned with matters of promotion, failure to hire, and discharge for discriminatory reasons. Sexual harassment charges are being heard more often than in the past. To date, however, such harassment is difficult to prove and to assess in relation to damages. Religious and ethical issues are continuing to arise in relation to job duties and scheduling. Issues of job segregation and wage discrimination are being widely publicized as issues of comparable worth.

Operating in a union-free environment or diminishing problems and expenses in a unionized setting requires careful attention to the issues inherent in discrimination. Title VII of the Civil Rights Act encouraged employees to seek remedies for discrimination. Legitimate complaints of flagrant abuses are so widespread that employers have become increasingly more cautious in terminating any employee. It is not unusual for discharged employees to play the game of "legal blackmail" by filing a charge with the EEOC or by filing a lawsuit for some act of alleged discrimination or for the so-called tort of wrongful discharge. These employees count on a hospital's desire to avoid bad publicity and the expense in money or time to fight the legal battle; they hope for a settlement. More and more employers are fighting such cases, however, to avoid setting a precedent.

The first concrete evidence that the prevalence of this problem has been recognized is the little known Equal Access to Justice Act, which became effective in October, 1981. This act permits small employers, individuals whose net worth is less than one million dollars, sole owners of businesses worth less than five million dollars, and businesses/associations/organizations with five hundred or fewer employees to hold government agencies responsible for part or all of their costs when the government's legal action is found to be substantially unjustified. Under this act, a federal agency that loses a case must show that its case was reasonably based on law and fact. If it cannot do so, the government agency will be responsible for all court-assigned costs.

Handling Charges of Employment Discrimination

Employment discrimination charges are harder to contend with today than ever before. Many charges may become class action suits, particularly in the areas of equal hiring, pay, and age discrimination. Such cases are being handled by the EEOC and the EEOC's new Early Litigation Identification (ELI) program.

The ELI program was created to review employee charges that were occupying a disproportionate amount of the EEOC's time. Before the ELI program was developed, EEOC investigators advocated individual remedies so often that a great backlog of cases accrued. Priority is now given to issues such as testing, failure to hire where there is existing underutilization, and failure to promote in circumstances of underutilization. The ELI program is also emphasizing the importance of identifying companies that have a low representation of minorities.[1]

As soon as a charge is filed, the employer should determine whether the charge involves any class action issues. The facts on company policy should be gathered. At times, the background information on a case is so voluminous that computers and statisticians are needed to handle the data. Employers are using such statistical proof more and more frequently when they must establish adequate utilization of a certain category of employee.

When the EEOC is investigating a charge, employers should discuss the breadth of the charge with the EEOC. It is also important to identify exactly which facility or department is involved in the charge.

Employers should limit the EEOC interviewing of employees. Although an employer is not required to allow an employee interview on company premises, a company representative can be present if the employer permits such an interview.

The EEOC should not have carte blanche to an employer's files unless the relevancy of certain disclosures can be established. Affirmative action documents and other equal opportunity materials should also be kept confidential unless their relevancy to a case is established. When employee files are reviewed by EEOC investigators, employee names may be deleted before the files are given to EEOC officials.

In complicated cases, both the government and the employer may submit position papers to clarify their facts and determinations in the case. Such position papers are also valuable to a judge who may have to review the case in court, but does not have the time to study the voluminous facts and statistical data necessary to an understanding of the case.

The hospital must decide at the outset whether to settle the case or to litigate it. Settlement is advisable when the hospital finds that the facts supporting its position are weak or when the potential impact on the hospital is classwide and serious doubt of the legality of the claim exists. In this situation, the company may opt for the predetermined settlement in which negotiations are confined to the charge. For example, in one case an elderly employee at the top of the pay scale who not only was lazy, but also had problems with alcohol and absenteeism was retired early as part of an economic cutback. This employee was made to view this "early retirement" as positive; after rethinking the issue, however, the employee filed a charge with the EEOC based on age discrimination. The employee had a strong case because of the employer's failure to make it clear if he was being retired, if he was being terminated for cause, or if he was merely being laid off as a result of the cutback. The employer settled the case by offering the employee another job, since it was rehiring at the time of case settlement. Pursuit of this charge in court would have embarrassed the employer, because the handling of the retirement had been less than optimal. In considering a hospital's legal course, the management team must evaluate the costs of litigation in time, money, energy, and other resources, as well as adverse publicity that might arise from litigation. A decision to litigate, however, might be wise if the hospital believes that settlement could establish an undesirable precedent.

Managers should realize that retaliation charges are becoming more common in EEOC cases. Now that the EEOC provides employers with a charge soon after it is filed, involved employees may interpret any action of their employer as one of retaliation and file a charge about such retaliatory treatment. When a case is pending before the EEOC, it is even more important to take consistent disciplinary action that is well founded in past practice, even when the employee provokes action deliberately.

Age Discrimination

In the 1980s, lawsuits based on age discrimination are becoming common.[2] The effects of inflation, difficult economic times, and the increasing mean age of the population are particularly felt in the health care industry because of its labor-intensive nature. When patient censuses drop and areas of hospitals are closed, plans are made for cutbacks. It soon becomes obvious that older workers are paid the most money even if they are not performing at the rate of a younger employee or keeping up with the rapid changes in health care.

The Age Discrimination in Employment Act, which prohibits discrimination in employment by employers, employment agencies, and labor organizations on the basis of age, was extended by Congress to include individuals from forty to seventy years of age. As a result of this act, employers may not discriminate against those in the protected age bracket in any terms, wages, retirement, conditions, or privileges of employment. Furthermore, notices of employment opportunities may not reflect age-related preferences, limitations, or specifications. (See *Kerwood v. Mortgage Bankers Association,* 494 F.Supp. 1298 23 EPD ¶ 31,043 [D.D.C. 1980]). This act also protects individuals who actively oppose age discrimination attempts against retaliation. Where two individuals between the ages of forty and seventy must be compared for a termination decision, age cannot be utilized as the basis for such a decision.

While the EEOC guidelines on the Age Discrimination Act are rather vague, once the protected individual has established a prima facie case, the burden of going forward for establishing factors of differentiation standards rests with the employer. Thus, a factor for employee differentiation that also has an adverse impact on employees in the protected age bracket must be justified and validated by the employer as a business necessity.

With respect to wage rate reductions, the EEOC's interpretation is less specific than that detailed by the Department of Labor, which formerly administered age discrimination matters. Employers now have more latitude in adjusting wage discrepancies. More importantly, the EEOC's guidelines allow for a broader interpretation of the law.

There have been lawsuits with negative outcomes for employers, however, in matters of age discrimination. In *Cancellier v. Federated Department Stores,* 28 FEP Cases 1151 (9th Cir. 1982), for example, three former executives of I. Magnin with a minimum of seventeen years experience won a total of $1.9 million in awards. This case exemplifies the potential liability of an employer in the area of age discrimination suits, since it involved a jury trial (to which an age discrimination plaintiff is entitled), punitive damages, and pendent state claims, such as the wrongful discharge claim.

Employers must carefully consider the matter of a jury trial, since juries not only assess case legality but also judge fairness. Jurors are inclined to be empathetic to an employee who has a record of lengthy, loyal service.

In these situations, the so-called "deep pocket" theory applies. Jurors consider companies better able to stand the loss of dollars than the individual. Thus, when the evidence indicates that the plaintiff has been unjustly treated by an employer's arbitrary termination of employment, jurors are inclined to vote in favor of the individual. Moreover, courts tend to be reluctant to overturn jury awards, even when the sympathy of the jurors' decision is obvious (see *Tribble v. Westinghouse Electric Corp.,* 669 F.2d 1193 [8th Cir. 1982]). In summary, plaintiff recoveries in age discrimination charges have included reinstatements; recovery of lost wages, pension, and other benefits; interest; and attorney's fees. While some cases have also involved start-up costs for beginning a new job or business, courts have varied in their awards for psychological damage, and pain and suffering.

Punitive damages have been awarded to plaintiffs when the employer has willfully violated the Age Discrimination Act. Such recoveries are generally twice the amount of the employee's lost earnings. While the definition of "willful violations" has been elusive, courts have generally focused on the employer's violation in terms of "knowing or voluntary" acts (see *Kelly v. American Standard, Inc.,* 640 F.2d 974, 980 [9th Cir. 1980]). In other cases such as *Wehr v. Burroughs Corp.,* 619 F.2d 276, 283 (3d Cir. 1980), simple disregard of the act by an employer was sufficient grounds for granting damages to the plaintiff. Discharge cases involving age discrimination can be expensive and awards can be high, since the time that elapses between the ADEA incident and the jury trial can be lengthy.

Pendent state claims may require proof similar to that required to show a violation of the Age Discrimination Act. Damages recovered can be quite different from state to state in individual cases, however. State statutes may provide relief for damage to a plaintiff's reputation or mental status.

DISCIPLINARY DECISIONS

The manager's right to discipline employees arises from employee obligations inherent in employment. Employment expectations expressed in policies and rules relate to the employee's duty to

1. be prepared and available to work during scheduled times
2. be appropriately fit to work
3. work productively
4. comply with personal, ethical, and professional standards of the health care delivery system
5. conform to appropriate behavioral standards
6. contribute to the client's and employer's well-being

Even though these six areas are well-developed in voluminous policy books, hospitals have serious problems in implementing disciplinary decisions, partly because of the inconsistent application of stated standards (see Chapter 9). Other problems arise from the legal difficulty of honestly applying disciplinary measures when equal employment opportunity is in question.

WRONGFUL DISCHARGE—TERMINATION AT WILL

Although the termination-at-will rule first appeared in a New York federal court case in 1849, it was 1908 before the Supreme Court ruled that either the employee or the employer could terminate the working relationship "for whatever reason" (*Adair v. United States,* 208 U.S. 161 [1908]). This right was based on the personal liberty intended in the Fifth Amendment to the Constitution.

Since the termination-at-will rule was purely stated at the turn of the century, a great deal has happened to constrain the employer's absolute rights. The National Labor Relations Act (NLRA) was enacted to protect the employees' right to engage or refrain from engaging in union organizing or protected concerted activities without loss of employment. Termination rights were further limited by the Civil Rights Act of 1964, the Age Discrimination in Employment Act, and the Vocational Rehabilitation Act for handicapped individuals. In *Whirlpool Corp. v. Marshall,* 100 S.Ct. 883 (1980), the Supreme Court upheld an Occupational Safety and Health Act regulation that provided that discipline for employee refusal to perform an act placing the employee in imminent danger is a violation of the Occupational Safety and Health Act.

The most explosive legal trend health care institutions face in the 1980s is the so-called tort of wrongful discharge or a discharge being found to be a violation of an implied contract, namely the hospital's handbook. There was an unsuccessful attempt in 1980 to enact a bill called the Corporate Democracy Act, introduced by Congressman Benjamin S. Rosenthal (D-N.Y.) and eight cosponsors. Title 4 of the bill, called Rights of Employees, was a proposal to amend the NLRA by stating that it was the policy of the United States to protect employees in the security of their employment by not permitting dismissal of an employee who had simply exercised a legal, civil, or constitutional right. This legislation provided that an employee could not be discharged unless *just cause* was found to exist. Criminal and civil penalties for corporations that violated this bill were also proposed.

Similar bills are pending in three states—Michigan, Pennsylvania, and Wisconsin—providing restrictions to the employer's common law right to discharge employees at will. Furthermore, Michigan recently passed a law that protects "whistle blowers," and South Dakota has a statutory restriction on the termination-at-will doctrine, providing that an employee who is hired at a yearly salary is presumed to be hired for a year and termination before the end of that year requires an employer to show that the termination resulted from a "habitual neglect of duty or continued incapacity to perform or any willful breach of duty by the employee."[3]

California has a statute that allows an employee hired for no specified term to be terminated at the will of either party on notice to the other; employment for a specified term is taken to mean employment for a period greater than one month. Montana has a statute enacted in 1885 that reinforces the common law doctrine that an employee hired for no specified term may be terminated at will.

The general rule has been that, if a hospital is not covered by a labor agreement that includes a "discharge only for cause" provision, the hospital can terminate an employee for any reason or even for no reason; when the employment is for an indefinite term, it is presumed to be a hiring at will, which may be freely terminated by either party at any time. As the highest court of the State of New York decided in *Murphy v. American Home Products,* 58 NY 2d 293, 461 NYS 2d 232, 448 NE 2d 86, 31 FEP CAS 782 (1983). "This Court has not and does not now recognize a cause of action in tort for abusive and wrongful discharge of an employee; such recognition must await action of the Legislature" (at 31 FEP CAS 782).

Erosion of the Termination-at-Will Doctrine

Termination of Employee for Refusal To Commit an Illegal Activity or Disclosing Illegal Activities

In our litigious society, the courts of different states have begun to erode the termination-at-will doctrine by allowing causes of action in tort to redress wrongful discharges. Thus, some states have recognized this tort and held employers liable for wrongful discharge when employees were dismissed in retaliation for conduct that is protected by the states' public policy. For example, wrongful termination has been found when employers have discharged employees for disclosing illegal activities on the part of their employers, such as antitrust violations, or whistle-blowing on an employer's intentional and deliberate marketing of unsafe products (see, e.g., *Sheets v. Teddy's Frosted Foods, Inc.,* 179 Conn. 471, 427 A.2d 385 [1980]; *Palmateer v. International Harvester Co.,* 85 Ill. 2d 124, 421 N.E.2d 876

[1981]; *Harless v. First National Bank,* 246 S.E.2d 270 [1978]; *Campbell v. Eli Lilly & Co.,* 413 N.E.2d 1054 [1980]); or for refusal to commit perjury (*Petermann v. International Brotherhood of Teachers,* 174 Cal. App. 2d 183, 344 P.2d 25 [1959]). In *Misecordia v. NLRB,* 104 LRRM 2666 (1980), for example, the employer attempted to fire a head nurse for engaging in protected concerted activity, namely, to inform the Joint Commission on Accreditation of Hospitals (JCAH) about certain deficiencies in the institution. In this case, the NLRA afforded the nurse protection, since she did not qualify as a supervisor under the act.

In *Perry v. Hartz Mountain Corporation,* 537 F. Supp. 1387 (USDC S.Ind., 1982), the District Court for the Southern District of Indiana held that, by alleging that Hartz discharged him for refusing to continue his participation in an illegal anticompetitive conspiracy, the plaintiff had stated a claim that fell within the exception to the employment-at-will doctrine. Courts have found other exceptions to the employment-at-will doctrine, such as employees who have been terminated because they have been called for jury duty (*Nees v. Hocks,* 277 Ore. 210, 536 P.2d 512 [1975]) or because they have filed worker's compensation claims (*Frampton v. Central Indiana Gas Co.,* 260 Ind. 249, 297 N.E.2d 425 [1973]; *Kelsay v. Motorola, Inc.,* 74 Ill. 2d 172, 384 N.E.2d 353 [1978]).

While there are a number of cases where courts have overturned a discharge on public policy grounds to protect the employee who informs official agencies of commissions or omissions that are not in the interest of the public, the following termination situations should be reviewed in order to have a complete picture of the doctrine of wrongful or negligent discharge.

The area of public policy as it relates to discharge involves some controversial ethical issues. There have been a number of cases that represent a clash of employee-employer interests when workers refuse to perform a job because of their moral objections. One case in the appeals process is *Kenny v. Ambulatory Centre of Miami,* 26 EPD ¶ 32,079 (Fla. 1981). In this case, a full-time operating room nurse was demoted to part-time status because of her refusal to participate in an abortion. According to Florida statute, this employee has the right to make such a refusal on religious grounds without suffering disciplinary action. The hospital must make reasonable efforts to implement alternative accommodations unless it would suffer undue hardship.

In another case, *Lamp v. Presbyterian Medical Center,* 590 P.2d 513 (Colo. App. 1978), a nurse was discharged for failing to comply with an order to reduce the staff in the intensive care unit to a level that would jeopardize patient care. Although the court in this case held that the general standard of conduct involving the health and safety of patients in the licensing statute did not provide the basis for a wrongful discharge action, other state court decisions show a trend toward carefully weighing differing standards and perspectives in ethical beliefs and behaviors. For example, in *Geary v. United States Steel Corp.,* 456 Pa. 171, 319 A.2d 174 (1974), the Pennsylvania Supreme Court upheld the decision of the lower court in allowing termination of employment because an employee had refused to sell a product that he believed to be defective. The court found that the employee did not have the credentials to determine matters of public safety. Although the employee action was sincere, it did not support a cause of action for wrongful discharge.

In *Hayes v. Shelby Memorial Hospital,* 30 EPD ¶ 33,058 (D.C. Ala. 1982), business necessity was found not to be a sufficient defense for the hospital's discharge of a radiation technologist in the second month of pregnancy. The hospital contended that it was concerned with the possible liability arising from fetal damage. The court ruled that, in view of the hospital's reluctance to allow the employee to continue taking radiographs and its inability to demonstrate that pregnancy was a hindrance to employment, the hospital was responsible for finding alternatives to discharge. In addition, a court of appeals has held that the alleged concern of a hospital that discharged a pregnant X-ray technician over the health of her fetus was a mere pretext for discrimination. (See *Zuniga v. Kleberg County Hospital* (Kingsville, Texas), (CA-5, 1982) 30 FEP CAS 650.)

In summary, the courts are finding themselves in the difficult position of deciding when employees may behave inconsistently within their normally stipulated employee role. They are being asked to determine whether sincere, honest employee actions should be honored because of the motive, even when the weight of the evidence does not support a cause for action. On the other hand, some consideration must be given to how much the courts can legislate in the affairs of hospitals and other businesses without interfering with the business' right to operate.[4] Because of the large number of women employed in health care facilities, pregnancy is a particular problem for hospitals.

In the case of *Gouveia v. Napili-Kai, Ltd.,* 65 Hawaii 189, 649 P.2d 1119 (1982), certification denied, (1983, U.S.) 103 S.Ct. 1873, the Supreme Court of Hawaii considered a state court tort action in which an employee claimed he had been wrongfully discharged because he attempted to engage in collective bargaining with his employer, the Napili-Kai Beach Club. Gouveia, who had been told by management that he was being paid union scale for his job, later claimed that his wage was below what those in unions made. When he sought to negotiate a higher wage for himself and other employees, he was terminated. Gouveia filed charges against the club with the National Labor Relations Board (NLRB), and a settlement was reached in which the club agreed to pay Gouveia two thousand dollars in back pay.

Six months later, Gouveia filed a state court lawsuit seeking general damages for deceit and negligent or intentional infliction of emotional distress, as well as punitive damages for malicious and outrageous conduct by the employer. He did not assert in state court the claims in his unfair labor practice charge and, in fact, asserted that the NLRB did not have jurisdiction to consider his claims of emotional distress resulting from the alleged outrageous conduct. When the case was appealed to the Hawaii Supreme Court, the justices dismissed it, holding that the claims were preempted by the NLRA and the NLRB as Gouveia was claiming that his discharge itself caused his mental distress, and the discharge also formed the basis of his unfair labor practice charge, which had been settled with the NLRB. The Hawaii Supreme Court held that something more than the mere act of discharge was needed for state court jurisdiction.

In seeking U.S. Supreme Court review, Gouveia contended that the Hawaii Supreme Court was wrong because the damages he sought could not have been awarded by the Board as he could not claim damages for mental distress in the NLRB administrative proceeding. The club, however, argued that review should be denied because the Board had accepted jurisdiction over the unfair labor practice charge and supervised its settlement. The U.S. Supreme Court refused to review the case.

In *Operating Engineers, Local 926 v. Jones*, 103 S.Ct. 1453 (1983, U.S.), the U.S. Supreme Court ruled that a wrongful discharge action in a state court, including a claim for punitive damages, is preempted by the NLRA, because the discharge of an employee as a result of a union's coercive conduct is actually prohibited by the Act. In the *Jones* case, although the NLRB assumed jurisdiction, the regional director refused to issue a complaint on the basis that there was "insufficient evidence" to show a violation of the NLRA. Even though there was no unfair labor practice administrative hearing on the charge, the Supreme Court decided that the regional director's refusal to issue a complaint was a decision covered by the preemption doctrine pointing to the supervisor's failure to exhaust his administrative remedy by appealing the regional director's decision to the NLRB General Counsel in Washington, D.C.

Further, if the basis of an employee's state or federal court complaint also would constitute an unfair labor practice under the NLRA, then the state or federal court must dismiss the complaint under the federal preemption doctrine. This is true even if the employee has not filed a charge to invoke the jurisdiction of the NLRB. This principle was recently upheld in *Buscemi v. McDonnell Douglas Corp.* (1982, C.D. Cal.), 113 LRRM 2788. A former employee of McDonnell-Douglas Corporation sued the company based on a California statute for wrongful discharge. The ex-employee claimed he was wrongfully discharged for "passing petitions among his fellow employees" and "voicing his objections as a spokesman for other employees concerning different personnel practices against the interests of the employees." The corporation filed a Motion to Dismiss, which was granted on the grounds that the court lacked subject-matter jurisdiction and that the ex-employee's complaint was within the exclusive jurisdiction of the NLRB, arguably protected and prohibited by Sections 7 and 8 of the NLRA and, therefore, preempted (citing *Magnuson v. Burlington Northern, Inc.*, 576 F.2d 1367 (9th Cir., 1978), *cert. denied*, 439 U.S. 930 (1978); *Columbia Power Trades Council v. U.S. Department of Energy*, 671 F.2d 325 (9th Cir., 1982)).

Therefore, even if an employee has not brought an unfair labor practice charge before the NLRB and the reason alleged for the discharge constitutes an unfair labor practice, the employee cannot successfully sue the hospital for wrongful discharge in state or federal court.

Also, in two recent cases, the termination-at-will doctrine was further eroded by judicial fiat broadening the concept of wrongful discharge. The Montana Supreme Court in *Gates v. Life of Montana Insurance Co.*, Mont. Sup. Ct. 162 DLR:A-7, E-1 (1983), held that the employer's "breach of the duty owed to deal fairly and in good faith which arises out of the employment relationship is a tort for which punitive damages may be imposed." The court upheld a jury award of $50,000 in punitive damages on the basis that the jury could infer from the testimony in the record that the plaintiff's supervisor told her he would give her a letter of recommendation if she resigned, without ever intending to do so. The supervisor said the letter would be returned to the plaintiff, while never intending to return it, all of which formed the basis for a jury finding of fraud, oppression, or malice, resulting in an award of punitive damages. There was a strong dissent warning that the majority's decision had "set the stage for a 'just cause standard for at-will employees,' which is a legislative rather than a judicial function."

In another termination-at-will case, the Nevada Supreme Court in *Southwest Gas Corporation v. Ahmad*, Nev. Sup. Ct. 176 DLR: A-5 (1983), held that the company's employee handbook was either a part of the original oral employment contract or a modification of it. In this case, the employee was discharged for unsatisfactory job performance and the provision in the handbook in question was that "termination for cause can occur only after notification from the employee's department head . . . of unsatisfactory performance." A sharply divided Nevada Supreme Court held that the employer breached its oral employment contract, as modified by the handbook, by discharging the employee without advance notice. Although the court concluded the employee was fired for cause, it found that she was entitled to damages for the employer's failure to follow the termination clause of the handbook.

A vigorous dissent rebuked the majority for "propelling Nevada law above and beyond those jurisdictions who have carefully engrafted limited exceptions" to the employment-at-will doctrine. The dissent, rightfully, in the authors' opinion, states that the handbook was no more than a "unilateral publication of the company policies and employee benefits," and warns that the majority ruling will cause employers to avoid publishing handbooks for fear of liability.

As shown by these two cases, if there is an employee handbook, follow it. Don't make any fraudulent misrepresentations at the exit interview. Deal with the terminated employee fairly, and be open and aboveboard. Treat them as individuals worthy of respect, particularly when disciplining or discharging them. In the case of terminating older employees, when the discharge procedure itself is handled abruptly and unfairly, a heavy-handed approach may tip the scales in favor of a lawsuit for wrongful discharge.

Tort of Outrage—Intentional Infliction of Emotional Harm

In *Vienstenz v. Fleming Companies, Inc.,* 681 F.2d 699 (CA-10, 1982) *cert. denied* (U.S. 1982) 95 LC ¶ 13,851, the Tenth Circuit Court of Appeals held that the conduct of the employer's security firm in questioning an employee, who later admitted to stealing merchandise and was discharged, was not so outrageous as to create an infliction of severe distress constituting the tort of outrage. The court held that such a claim would conflict with federal regulation of labor disputes under the Labor Management Relations Act, 1947.

In *Vienstenz,* the employee brought suit in U.S. District Court charging the employer with wrongful discharge and also with the tort of outrage for infliction of emotional distress—a claim that was allowed by the district court to go to a jury trial. Vienstenz testified in the lower court action that he admitted to the theft only because of fear of losing his job and that his subsequent discharge caused him worry and fright. A federal jury awarded him more than $50,000 in damages, later reduced by the district court to $25,000 in punitive damages and $2,500 in actual damages.

While the Tenth Circuit agreed with the lower court in dismissing the wrongful discharge claim, it overturned the lower court on the outrage claim stating that the distress suffered by Vienstenz stemmed from his discharge and not the interview itself and, therefore, was a case preempted by the NLRB's jurisdiction. The court further held that even if the distress stemmed from the interview, the conduct of the employer's security firm was not sufficiently outrageous.

To further constitute the tort of outrage, the employer's conduct must be so outrageous and extreme as to go beyond all possible bounds of decency and be regarded as atrocious and utterly intolerable in a civilized community (*Novosel v. Sears, Roebuck & Co.,* 495 F.Supp. 344 (E.D. Dist. Ct. Mich. 1980)).

Exhibit 10-1 is an actual complaint (with fictitious names) that was filed in a state court. It alleges that the wrongful discharge violated the plaintiff's constitutional rights, her state and federal rights, and the public policy of the state; furthermore, it claims that the written disciplinary report resulting in her discharge was false and defamatory. The wrongful discharge features of this complaint (not the defamation allegations) would be preempted by the NLRA and dismissed by state court on the appropriate motion to dismiss.

If the written Employee Disciplinary Report of which the plaintiff complained in Counts IV and V of Exhibit 10-1 was not false, but was in fact true, the question becomes whether the hospital can defame an employee by alleging improper and defective performance by an employee in a written disciplinary report drawn up pursuant to the hospital's policies and procedures. In the case of *Louisville & N. R.*

Exhibit 10–1 Sample Complaint of Wrongful Discharge

WASHINGTON CIRCUIT COURT
CIVIL ACTION NO. 0000000
DIVISION No. 1

MARY R. JONES   PLAINTIFF
v.   COMPLAINT
GOOD SAMARITAN HOSPITAL   DEFENDANT

Comes now the Plaintiff, Mary R. Jones, and for her complaint states as follows:

PARTIES

A. Plaintiff, Mary R. Jones, is a resident of Washington County in Your State.
B. Defendant, Good Samaritan Hospital, is a not-for-profit institution in Your State. Its registered office is in Your State at 3212 Main Street, Smithville, Your State.

COUNT I

1. Plaintiff is employed by Good Samaritan Hospital and has been an employee at said company for eight years as a licensed practical nurse. Plaintiff's employment was terminated by the defendant on or about June 28, 1982.
2. Plaintiff's duties consisted primarily of providing nursing care under the direction of a registered nurse and in compliance with the policies, rules, licensing restrictions, and job description of said position.
3. During the fall and winter of 1981, plaintiff and her co-workers actively participated in and supported an attempted unionization effort of licensed practical nurses at Good Samaritan Hospital.
4. Plaintiff's participation in and support of the unionization of defendant hospital was known to the management and officers of defendant hospital.
5. Plaintiff's employment was terminated by defendant employer on June 28, 1982. Said termination of plaintiff was planned in advance and was in retaliation for plaintiff's activity in supporting the unionization of defendant hospital.
6. Plaintiff states that defendant's actions constituted a wrongful termination of plaintiff's employment.
7. As a result of defendant's wrongful acts, plaintiff's reputation in the community has been damaged; she has suffered loss of wages, and she has endured mental suffering and emotional distress. Plaintiff has been damaged in the sum of $100,000.

COUNT II

8. Plaintiff readopts, realleges, and incorporates by reference herein all the allegations contained in Count I of plaintiff's complaint.
9. The termination of plaintiff's employment from defendant corporation was in retaliation for plaintiff's exercise of her right of freedom of speech and freedom of association as protected under the First Amendment to the Constitution of the United States.
10. Plaintiff states that defendant's actions constituted a wrongful termination of plaintiff's employment and were contrary to the public policy of this state.
11. As a result of defendant's wrongful acts, plaintiff's reputation in the community has been damaged; she has suffered loss of wages; and she has endured mental suffering and emotional distress. Plaintiff has been damaged in the sum of $100,000.

Exhibit 10–1 continued

COUNT III

12. Plaintiff readopts, realleges, and incorporates by reference herein all the allegations contained in Counts I and II of the complaint.
13. The termination of plaintiff's employment was in violation of federal and state statutes and the United States Constitution. Pursuant to XRS 446.070, plaintiff hereby claims damages as hereafter stated.
14. As a result of defendant's wrongful act, plaintiff's reputation in the community has been damaged; she has suffered loss of wages; and she has endured mental suffering and emotional distress. Plaintiff has been damaged in the sum of $100,000.

COUNT IV

15. Plaintiff readopts, realleges, and incorporates by reference herein all the allegations contained in Counts I, II, and III of plaintiff's complaint.
16. On or about June 28, 1982, an employee of Good Samaritan Hospital prepared an "Employee Disciplinary Report" in regard to plaintiff's job performance.
17. The report was prepared by an employee of the defendant at the direction of officers and management of defendant corporation.
18. Said report was used as the basis to terminate plaintiff's employment. Further, said report meant and was understood to mean by persons reading said report that plaintiff's work was defective and improper; that she was a poor employee and failed to follow the policy of her employer.
19. The information contained in said report is false and defamatory.
20. At the time said report was prepared, defendant hospital's employees and officers knew that the statements contained in said report were untrue and were made for the sole purpose of providing a subterfuge under which plaintiff's employment could be terminated. Defendant's officers and employees, in making said report, were acting in the course of their employment; and were acting with malice and in reckless disregard of the truth.
21. As a result of said defamatory statements, plaintiff's reputation in the community has been damaged; she has suffered loss of wages; and she has endured mental suffering and emotional distress. Plaintiff has been damaged in the sum of $100,000.

COUNT V

22. The wrongful acts and defamatory statements above referred to were intentional and were activated with actual malice and willful intent to injure plaintiff in the manner as set forth above. Therefore, plaintiff is entitled to punitive damages in the sum of $100,000.

WHEREFORE, plaintiff demands as follows:
1) Judgment against defendant for compensatory damages in the amount of $400,000, and punitive damages in the sum of $100,000;
2) Interest thereon at the legal rate;
3) Costs herein expended;
4) Trial by jury; and
5) Any and all other relief to which plaintiff may be entitled.

> SMITH & SMITH
> 123 State Street
> Smithville, Your State
> ATTORNEYS FOR PLAINTIFF

Co. v. Marshall 586 S.W.2d 274 (1979), the Kentucky Court of Appeals considered a state libel action brought by a former employee who claimed that the conduct of his supervisor in preparing written statements critical of the former employee's work was libelous. The court held that such statements critical of the employee's work were not outrageous conduct as these statements were not published to anyone within the company who did not have a legitimate interest in the subject matter of such statements. Therefore, the statements were privileged communications under the terms of the collective bargaining agreement. The Kentucky Court of Appeals, in finding such statements privileged, stated at 586 S.W.2d 282, 283, "In the instant case, the only publication of this report was to the secretary who typed the reports and to those supervisory employees with a 'legitimate interest in the subject matter.'" Thus, following established disciplinary procedures pursuant to a formal disciplinary system and publishing critical remarks only to those supervisory personnel who have a legitimate interest in the subject matter, may exculpate an employer from a defamation charge. A Massachusetts district court found that a company's designation on a personnel form that the terminated employee was a "minor loss" and that it would not rehire the employee does not constitute defamation. The court found that the company was entitled to its opinions and the statement was made on a routine internal communication intended solely for those management officials with a "need to know." (See *Underwood v. Digital Equipment Corp. Inc.,* U.S.D.C. Mass. 226 DLR: A-1 (1983).) Also, the court found that the employee's claim of emotional distress based on alleged harassment due to race discrimination was barred by Massachusetts workers' law.

If the written disciplinary report referred to in Exhibit 10-1 was in fact false, the same principle is used; if the disciplinary report is published only pursuant to an official disciplinary system, such as those contemplated by a collective bargaining agreement, and published only to those with a legitimate interest in the subject matter, it may not be made the subject of a defamation or libel action. There are cases that offer guidance on this point. In the case of *Joftes v. Kaufman,* 324 F. Supp. 660, 662 (D.D.C. 1971), for example, the court stated:

> All these arguments point in the direction of one principle: That notices of dismissal for cause which are contemplated by a collective bargaining agreement and which are published by the employer only to those with a legitimate interest in the subject matter may not be made the subject of an action in libel, *regardless of whether the allegations of cause are true or false and regardless of the actual motive behind the dismissal.* This principle finds ample support in the law and requires that summary judgment be entered for defendants as to each cause of action. (Emphasis supplied.)

*Termination for Violating a Written Employer Policy As Contained in
Employer's Handbook*

The employee handbook and policy manual further define employee rights, since
in some states they are considered an implied contract with the employee. In the
case of *Weiner v. McGraw-Hill,* 57 N.Y.2d 458, 457 N.Y.S.2d 193, 443 N.E.2d
441 (1982), the New York Court of Appeals upheld the right of an employee of the
defendant to sue the publishing firm for firing him without the "just and sufficient
cause" mandated in the employer's personnel handbook. The court found that the
personnel handbook was an employment contract and that the company breached
the contract by terminating the employee without cause. The court rejected
McGraw-Hill's argument that an oral promise of job security given the employee
when he was hired was in no way binding on the company.

The general rule that employment arrangements having no definite duration
constitute contracts-at-will terminable by either party has been eroded. An employer's written policy providing for discharge only for cause may become a part of
an indefinite term contract based upon the employee's legitimate expectations
generated by the employer's written statements (*Toussaint v. Blue Cross and Blue
Shield,* 408 Mich. 579, 292 N.W.2d 880 [1980]).

Thus, there is a growing body of opinion from labor law experts making the case
for employers who want to operate in a union-free environment to call their
handbooks employment contracts and provide for discharge only for cause,
enabling the hospital to counter the union argument that a labor contract is needed
for job security.

Prevention of Wrongful Termination Charges

All written policies, particularly those in an employee handbook, should be
followed strictly, especially as they pertain to terminations. Employers should
devise a system that keeps them up-to-date, as the law on wrongful discharges
evolves rapidly.

Prevention of wrongful discharge liability begins at the initial preemployment
interview. Interviewers must not make specific promises concerning job security,
"permanent employment," or training and advancement. Oral representations
concerning a worker's employment duration status should be avoided. Employee
handbooks should not guarantee any length of employment and should not limit
terminations to those for "just cause" unless the hospital has made a decision to call
it a contract as discussed earlier. In fact, employers should review their employee
handbook and job application forms to ensure that they do not contain terms
implying permanent employment or job security. Rather than the words *annual
salary* or *permanent,* terms such as *full-time, part-time,* or *regular* employee
should be used. It should be stated somewhere in all job application forms and

employee handbooks that employment is at will subject to termination at any time by either party, and that policies may be changed with or without notice by the employer at any time.

An employer must also realize that courts, like arbitrators, favor progressive disciplinary systems and that all employer disciplinary actions must be consistent and documented. Even oral disciplinary warnings should be noted in an employee's file.

With the erosion of the employment-at-will doctrine, some employers may want to make a written individual employment agreement spelling out the employment relationship. Such individual agreements limit an employer's flexibility, however, and may not cover a given discharge situation in the future. Also, they create an additional administrative burden if they are not updated to incorporate changes in hospital policy. In using a written individual employment agreement, an employer should consider the termination provision for both parties, compensation packages, job duties, notice requirements, and job performance expectations.

In a wrongful discharge/negligent termination case even where the hospital has cause for the discharge, it could be claimed that the employer may still be liable for failure to warn the employee of defective conduct or for the employer's failure to follow the system of performance appraisals.

Further, to avoid having the terminated employee returning to the hospital, give the ex-employee all benefits, such as vacation pay, at the time of discharge (even though it could be argued that the employee was not entitled to such benefits). Giving the ex-employee the benefits immediately may keep him from filing a wrongful discharge claim.

Exit interviews should be used to elicit any admissions the employee has concerning his discharge. A witness should be present and should take notes.

REDUCTION IN FORCE

Until recently, the term "reductions in force" (RIFs) was more common in the military services. Because of hard economic times, however, the term of RIF has become more frequent among white collar workers even in the health care industry.

One of the first approaches that employers consider when a RIF is necessary is involuntary retirement of more highly paid, older workers. In *McMann v. United Air Lines,* 542 F.2d 217 (CA-4, 1976) 12 EPD ¶ 11,209, reversed and remanded (U.S. 1977) 434 U.S. 192, the court found that involuntary retirement of employees within the group protected by the Age Discrimination Act was permissible only when legitimate factors other than age could be cited. The Supreme Court ruled that an employee could be retired because of age if it was done in accordance with a bona fide pension plan that was in effect prior to the enactment of the Age

Discrimination Act. Subsequently, Congress reviewed the intent of the act and amended it to prohibit new or existing plans allowing involuntary retirement.

Employers should beware of attempts to force older workers from the work force by citing inadequate training. In *Coates v. National Cash Register Co.*, 433 F. Supp. 655 (W.D. Va. 1977), the court's decision not to uphold such a discharge was based on an investigation that showed a relationship between employee training and age. Training practices and records of such activities caused the court to consider this case an Age Discrimination Act violation. Employers should also be careful not to attempt to defend a RIF on the basis of who can adjust to the new management style, who is the most qualified, and other factors that cannot be proved.

In instituting voluntary retirement actions, employers must ensure that the employee has not been directly or indirectly coerced into such a decision. The involved employee should be asked to sign a statement of understanding about the provisions of the termination agreement and the voluntary election of such a procedure (see *Ackerman v. Diamond Corp.*, 670 F.2d 66 [6th Cir. 1982]). In addition to obtaining the employee's signature, the hospital should make every effort to assist the new retiree in seeking another job or adjusting to retirement. Such assistance would be viewed favorably by a court hearing future claims on the action. If incentives are offered as part of a voluntary retirement package, deadlines should be established for the offer. Otherwise, employees who wish to retire when the hospital is enjoying normal economic times might be able to file a claim to similar benefits.

In reducing the force by discharging salaried employees who are not covered by the NLRA because of their supervisory status, employers should carefully consider potential wrongful discharge claims in relation to Title VII of the Civil Rights Act as well as claims under other state civil rights acts and claims under the Age Discrimination Act. For a plaintiff to substantiate a claim of wrongful discharge because of age discrimination when a RIF has occurred, the claimant must demonstrate

1. membership in the protected group
2. qualifications that would permit the claimant to work in another capacity at the institution
3. adverse impact resulting from the employer's action
4. employer intent to discriminate on the basis of age

Proof of the fourth criterion requires evidence of willful, purposeful discrimination by the employer in relation to the claimant's age.

Plan

Because RIFs will be a particular challenge to hospitals in the coming decade, administrators will need to approach them honestly and systematically, while minimizing legal liability. While no plan can ensure the employer complete protection from litigation, a planned approached to RIF is prudent.

The successful RIF begins with a careful review of the philosophy, mission, and objectives of the hospital in light of economic and other resource realities. Contingency plans for periods of financial distress should be formulated *prior* to any such crisis so that they can be implemented in an orderly way when the need arises. The plan should provide minimal to drastic steps. First steps may include avoiding temporary or permanent layoffs through such measures as an across the board reduction in pay, a rotating system for taking days off without pay, or no replacement of employees lost through attrition. In establishing the right plan, hospital managers must remember that the manner in which such measures are implemented can be subjected to the judgment of jurors, as well as to that of other agencies and professionals in the health care industry. The need for such action may not be questioned as much as the orderliness and fairness of the action to involved employees. A reputation for fairness is an important asset in attracting qualified physicians and health care workers, as well as clients, to a health care agency.

Cutbacks in the health care industry present problems that are not typical in other business settings. For example, factory line shutdowns might result in the production of fewer parts, whereas personnel cutbacks in hospitals might cause patients to suffer irreparable physical or mental damage; cardiac arrests cannot be programmed to occur only when staffing is adequate. Moreover, holistic care is not totally quantifiable. Time spent motivating a patient to live and swallow liquids evades mathematical formulations.

Justification

Because courts require employers to justify RIF decisions in litigation, employers must have a defensible rationale for their actions. Hospitals are taking a hard look at issues of productivity as they wrestle with the need to provide cost-effective health care services.[5] In evaluating staffing and productivity patterns, hospitals need to consider the following points:

1. What formulas can be computerized to allow simple, continuous feedback on the level of care required by the in-house patient population?
2. How can an equitable charge be formulated to assess users for the appropriate costs of nursing services, such as allaying a patient's fear of dying, giving a needed bath to a patient who refused the bath because of the inability to pay, services rendered when the patient is marginally competent to decide on the necessity of such services?
3. What can be done to provide the kind of professional help required by an aging population and to meet needs related to the extraordinary bio-

psychological outcomes of the technological and medical revolution that prolongs the lives of those with profound health problems?

4. What can hospitals do to cooperate with each other in avoiding duplication of poorly staffed and underutilized services while remaining competitive as a business during a RIF?

5. How can the RIF be managed so that sufficient numbers of qualified staff effectively meet surges in the patient load? Should cross-training programs be established to allow floating of staff and the proper mix of professional and ancillary staff?

6. How can hospital services be better marketed to attract a variety of patients who can pay more promptly for services rendered? How can more profitable services be better utilized to offset the costs of those that break even or lose money?

If, after all prudent measures for cost containment and efficient resource utilization have been implemented and documented, personnel cutbacks are still warranted, hospital managers must ensure that evidence supports the action on the basis of undisputable business necessity. They must be prepared to demonstrate the logic behind the plans of cutbacks, transfers, and layoffs.

Management Training

When a RIF is imminent, the top administrators need to plan a thoughtful strategy that involves all department heads, because the managers' commitment to the plan and support of the hospital are essential for smooth implementation of any RIF efforts. One example where this was *not* done is as follows:

XYZ Hospital took a head-in-the-sand approach to staff cutbacks. As census levels dropped below budgeted levels, the anxiety of the senior officers rose greatly. Still publicly optimistic, senior executives "quietly" closed a wing and circulated a voluntary form for cutbacks, wherein benefits and positional rights would continue through this "temporary request." Expenditures were tightly monitored and permissions for relief help were unilaterally squelched even when the need was justifiable. Staff discussed their insecurity with the top managers, who seemed to be rushing to put out brushfires without a game plan. Since the actions of the administrators spoke louder than their words, employees began to worry about the general status of the hospital. With widespread layoffs in the area, spouses became concerned. Employees began to interpret stray comments and isolated decisions as signs of doom and gloom. Worried employees confronted middle managers, who were also receiving mixed signals. The middle managers responded by being angry at top administrators because of their embarrassment over being excluded. As the credibility gap grew between top management and others in the hospital, numerous problems occurred in communication. Anxieties increased, tempers flared, and middle managers reinforced the registered nurses in bringing in a union.

To avoid such problems, the hospital management team should take care to communicate to all the need for a RIF and to allow constructive input from all participants. For reasons of business continuity and legalities, it is essential to explain to managers how to communicate this information to employees. A key aspect of a RIF should be an effort to find displaced employees other jobs in the institution or to assist them in finding comparable employment elsewhere. While assistance in other placement is not legally required, it is an important plus for public relations and for future litigation. Other jobs in the institution should be offered to the employee who is qualified, when possible.

In setting the policies that govern the RIF program, managers need to determine the actual monetary savings after the cost of the program implementation and potential legal liabilities have been calculated. In anticipation of potential legal liability from a RIF, the hospital should evaluate the cutbacks and what effect they will have due to an employee's age, race, sex, nationality, and union activities or lack thereof.

Communication

Because a swift dispatch of correct information is critical to avoid undesirable behaviors as a reaction to rumors, an early part of a RIF program must be an honest, clear explanation of the hospital's financial status to all employees in both written and oral form. The best person to provide this explanation is the chief executive officer. The importance of consistency in such reporting cannot be overemphasized. Every member of the management team should have the same information to disseminate at the same time. In times of a RIF, daily talks should be implemented so that middle managers remain up-to-date on the situation (see Chapter 8).

Some top administrators worry about information leaks when all department heads are aware of plans. Such worries are often justified. In anticipation of such security leaks, top managers should be prepared to move swiftly after the notification of middle management to the dissemination of information to all employees. The place for secrecy is in the data collection and formulation phase of the plan— not in the implementation stage. In the haste of the implementation, middle management input must be sought and utilized; otherwise, the plan may be sabotaged.

When a RIF program is announced, a freeze on hiring is appropriate. Older employees should be told that they will be given preference for available jobs if their area or division is cut back or closed. The hospital's thrust in the public relations effort at this time should be in emphasizing loyalty to its employees and in advertising continuity of services to the public.

Implementation

Once the mechanics of a RIF program have been determined, the most difficult aspect must be faced. Managers must confront individuals with bad news. Poor performers whose efforts have gone uncorrected are the most likely candidates for these termination interviews, which typically occur at the close of the work week. Older employees who have not kept their skills up-to-date and whose productivity has diminished often fall in this target population. It is advisable to have another manager present during the termination interview so that there is no mistake as to what was said.

An alternative approach works well in hospitals facing RIFs. A RIF committee, comprised of five members of the hospital staff who represent diverse interests such as older members, females, and minorities, may be vested with the authority to make decisions about who is to be removed or transferred. The committee approach has the advantage of providing not only a more objective means of decision making, but also a readily available source of witnesses for any litigations in the future. Members of the committee review the abilities, skills, and length of service of employees in relation to the needs of the hospital. To assist committee members in making personnel decisions, the director of personnel may be included as a nonvoting member of the committee.

After receiving an orientation to their functions, the committee members should adopt an evaluation tool that can be used to assess each hospital employee in relation to the RIF. Then, department heads make the comparable evaluations of employees in their departments and prepare to meet with the committee to make recommendations on employees to the committee. The personnel director, head nurses, or appropriate others may add detailed data to help the committee make RIF determinations. Expected reduction levels should then be stated so that the number of affected employees can be identified.

Termination seems to allow a hospital to remain more flexible than does a layoff with a recall option. Decisions on terminations should require unanimous approval of the committee. The supporting evidence of each committee member should be added to the decision. If a unanimous decision cannot be reached, those dissenting should place their reasons for their dissent in writing. The termination process should be supportive to the employee involved. Employees affected by the RIF should be allowed to appear before the committee in their own behalf and to bring others that want to speak for them. Through the use of a RIF committee, data may be presented to support the decision for termination. Such a decision is more defensible than a decision made by one person, who may later be shown to have some personal bias against the affected party.

The RIF committee may become involved in voluntary retirement proceedings if the hospital encourages employees to elect voluntary retirement. It may be prudent for the hospital to have a written record of all questions and answers that were discussed in counseling sessions on the retirement. The document to effect the voluntary retirement should have his reasons for electing early retirement and should be signed only when the employee has had two or three meetings with managers and adequate time to make an unpressured decision. It is also wise to allow a fifteen-day period in which the employee can revoke the decision to retire. An important case in the area of whether the retirement is actually voluntary is *Ackerman v. Diamond Corp.,* 670 F.2d 66 (CA-6, 1982).

Many hospitals are becoming part of larger corporations. In any merger, all factors related to the discharge of employees who cannot be placed in the new organization must be carefully reviewed and documented. Care should be taken to abide by statements in the employee handbook, since they may remain in force even when the new organization takes charge. Alterations in the work force should be meticulously handled so that a defensible position is established for any subsequent legal actions.

The Successful RIF

The first step in assessing changes that need to be made is for staff members and managers, working together, to separate essential functions from desirable and deletable tasks. As a result of this collaboration, some work may be consolidated or eliminated.

The next step for the RIF is to select an evaluation process for employees. When the criteria for the RIF are established, issues such as the consideration of seniority should be resolved so that a uniform standard may be applied to all employees. Records that have been kept according to the behavioral objectives method are one good means of providing more objective data on which to base judgment.

Because the termination rankings of the middle manager may not be consistent with prior performance appraisals, directors need to review and resolve any discrepancies. When prior performance appraisals have indicated that an employee worked well, but the same individual was selected for termination, subsequent lawsuits have proved embarrassing for the employer (see *Kephart v. Institute of Gas Technology,* 630 F.2d 1217 [7th Cir. 1980]).

Next is the exit interview. Two hospital managers should be present at each exit interview. Extraneous comments about age, sex, or retirement should be avoided, as innocent comments may be taken out of context in any future discrimination charge. The terminated employee has the right to an explanation of how employees for termination were compared with others, why his or her job was eliminated, and why he or she has been selected to leave the organization. The employee should be given the opportunity to ask questions related to this action.

The RIF process is a time-consuming process that must be well planned and executed to protect the interests of the hospital, its staff, and the public. When management does not take the time to consider this important move carefully, disastrous legal outcomes may result (see *Franci v. Avco Corp, Avco Lycoming Division*, 18 EPD ¶ 8789 (D.C. Ct. 1978). The RIF process is summarized in Exhibit 10-2.

COMPARABLE WORTH

Comparable worth is a recent legal theory under Title VII of the 1964 Civil Rights Act used to prove sex discrimination in wages. In applying this doctrine, employees compare their wages to those of other workers performing dissimilar jobs to establish Title VII pay violations. Under comparable worth, employees argue that different classes of jobs are undervalued because traditionally they have been segregated by sex. However, courts have been reluctant to uphold comparable worth claims unless the employees who claim discrimination prove they have substantially comparable and identical job skills. This theory also holds that even though the employees are arguing equal pay violations through sex discrimination under Title VII, the cases must be free of the equal work standard of the Equal Pay Act, which doesn't cover the more subtle forms of sex discrimination in wages. Under the comparable worth theory of the Equal Pay Act, employees file Title VII sex-based wage discrimination actions against employers based on a comparison of the value of similar but not identical jobs having the same comparable worth to the hospital.[6-10]

In *County of Washington v. Gunther* (U.S. S.Ct. 1981), 101 S.Ct. 2242, 25 FEP Cases 1521, the U. S. Supreme Court in a five to four decision, held that women employees who claimed that their jobs were undervalued because of intentional sex discrimination could proceed with their lawsuit under Title VII, even though they did not perform work identical to that required of male coworkers. The Court rejected the employer's argument that the suit should be dismissed because it did not meet the equal pay for equal work standard set forth in the Equal Pay Act. While the Supreme Court stressed that its ruling did not address the comparable worth issue, it did hold that claims for sex-based wage discrimination can be brought under Title VII even though no member of the opposite sex holds an equal but higher-paying job, provided that the challenged wage rate is not based on seniority, merit, quantity, or quality of production, or any other factor other than sex (namely, the four affirmative defenses authorized by the Equal Pay Act).

Exhibit 10–2 Summary of Reductions-in-Force (RIF) Programs

I. Plan
  - Review the philosophy, mission and objectives of the hospital in light of economic and resource realities.
  - Incorporate survival strategy into qualitative aspects of health care.
  - Write the plan into phases divided into minimal, moderate or maximum intervention, as based on the nature of the crisis.
  - Select a fair and orderly method for implementing each portion of the program.
  - Identify the requisite public relations efforts that will be necessary with clients, employees, suppliers, and other publics.
  - Prepare press releases and other materials that could be updated and rapidly distributed when the program is implemented.
  - Plan the strategy for communicating the RIF to physicians.

II. Justification
  - Prepare documents to show how the hospital has taken all steps to operate in a cost effective manner prior to and concurrent with the RIF.
  - Study the planned action in relation to protected groups under EEO guidelines, so that all actions taken can be legally defensible.
  - Gather quantitative data on productivity, staffing patterns, acuity, census, and job analyses.
  - Evaluate programs instituted on cross training and staff utilization. Review the staffing mix of professional and ancillary workers and justify recommendations.
  - Provide explicit objectives to show how the education department contributed to employee awareness and effectiveness in wise resource utilization.
  - Make recommendations based on *business necessity* which show the logic and rationale underlying the cutbacks, transfers, and discharges inherent in your RIF plan.

III. Management Training
  - Encourage all department heads to contribute ideas to the RIF plan as presented by top management.
  - Secure the commitment of all hospital managers to this plan through encouraging participation, and through a thorough presentation of the factual situation.
  - Educate the managers in the business and legal implications of the plan.
  - Outline the plan for informing all employees.
  - Be certain that all managers understand the plan, the justification for its implementation, and the information that employees will have on the plan.
  - Emphasize the importance of assisting employees to find other employment and the general public relations effort.

Exhibit 10–2 continued

IV. Communication
- Present a consistent, factual account of information on RIF.
- Utilize "Daily Talks" to keep middle managers and employees updated on the situation.
- Announce a hiring freeze.
- Simultaneously announce the RIF program and how it will affect employees.
- Publicize loyalty to employees and continuity of patient care services as a priority.

V. Implementation
- Determine who will be involved.
- Document performance.
- Confront employees and document termination interviews.
- Assist displaced employees in finding other employment.

In *Gunther,* four female prison guards brought suit under Title VII claiming that their employer had illegally set their pay at 70 percent of the rate paid to male guards, even though the employer's job evaluation study indicated that they should have been paid at 95 percent of the men's rate. The women insisted that the employer's failure to pay them the evaluated wage rate was the result of intentional sex discrimination. The women did not contend, the court noted, that they were entitled to "increased compensation on the basis of a comparison of the intrinsic worth or difficulty of their job with that of other jobs in the same organization or community." Instead, the court said, they are seeking to prove that they are victims of intentional sex discrimination, consisting of the employer's "setting the wage scale for female guards, but not for male guards, at a lower level than its own survey of outside markets and the worth of the jobs warranted."

The court noted that the women's right to sue under Title VII depended on whether the Bennett Amendment to Title VII incorporates the Equal Pay Act's equal pay for equal work standard, or only the Equal Pay Act's four affirmative defenses as noted previously. The Bennett Amendment provides that an employer may differentiate on the basis of sex in determining compensation if "such differentiation is authorized" by the Equal Pay Act. The court held that the Bennett Amendment incorporates only the four affirmative defenses of the Equal Pay Act into Title VII, and not the entire equal work standard. To hold that intentional sex-based wage discrimination only violated Title VII if it also violated the Equal Pay Act "means that a woman who is discriminatorily underpaid could obtain no relief—no matter how egregious the discrimination might be—unless her employer also employed a man in an equal job in the same establishment at a higher rate of pay. The court further pointed out that the County of Washington's interpretation of the Bennett Amendment would deny the right of women holding jobs not equal to those held by men proving that the system is a pretext for discrimination where the employer is using a transparently sex-biased system for wage determination.

The leading case dealing with the theory of comparable worth in the health care field is *Lemons v. City and County of Denver,* 620 F.2d 228 (CA-10, 1980), 22 FEP Cases 959, where nurses working for the city started at $1,000 less than painters, tree trimmers, and tire servicemen. These nurses battled to make their salaries equal to those general service categories rather than equal to those of other low-paid community nurses. The court held that the pay disparity claim was not seeking equality of opportunity for their skills as contemplated by Title VII, but was a claim of comparable worth where the nurses wanted the court to compare their jobs with jobs of entirely different skills. Such actions would open up "a whole new world for the courts," and the courts should not venture into such a world until "some better signal from Congress is received" (620 F.2d at 229). The Supreme Court denied certiorari (U.S. S.Ct. 1980) 449 U.S. 888, 23 FEP Cases 1668.

Another important case is *Briggs v. City of Madison* (U.S.D.C. Wis. 1982), 28 FEP Cases 793. Female public health nurses were paid less than male public health sanitarians, and thus claimed sex discrimination since the male public health sanitarians performed jobs requiring the same or a lesser degree of qualifications, skill, effort, and responsibility under similar working conditions. The public health nurses provide nursing services in emergency health situations for public schools, private homes, satellite offices; operate health clinics, including special immunization clinics; disseminate health education information; and perform a variety of other health related functions. The sanitarians had similar educational requirements and their responsibilities included inspecting eating and drinking establishments, retail food stores, hotels and motels, pools and beaches for compliance with applicable health rules and regulations; inspecting schools for compliance with safety rules and regulations; reviewing plans for private sewage systems and responding to complaints concerning sewage systems; investigating reports of food-borne illness and environmental complaints; and providing services at health clinics, including special immunization clinics; and providing assistance in emergency health situations, as well as other health related duties.

The court held that the nurses did not make a prima facie case as their approach did not eliminate the most common nondiscriminatory reason for wage disparity— the differences in the jobs' requirements of skill, effort, and responsibility. The City of Madison also showed that it had much more difficulty in attracting qualified sanitarians and that much of the continuing pay differential was derived from a survey conducted by a consulting firm. The public nurses claimed that the defendant could not use market conditions as a defense for upgrading the pay ranges of male sanitarians and not the public health nurses. This argument was based on the premise that the market reflects the biases and stereotypes of the value of women's work and, in particular, reflects the devaluation of nurses' salaries resulting from female domination of the nursing field. But the court held that under Title VII an employer's liability extends only to its own acts of discrimination.

The court stated that "nothing in the Act indicates that the employer's liability extends to conditions of the marketplace which it did not create; that there may be an abundance of applicants qualified for some jobs and a dearth of skilled applicants for other jobs is not a condition for which a particular employer bears responsibility." The nurses argued that case law supported the contention that employers cannot justify wage disparities between males and females performing equal work by asserting the greater difficulty of recruiting men for these jobs. The court stated that the decisions cited are not applicable to a case like this where not essentially identical skills are required for both jobs at issue, but rather that the kinds of skills are closely related and that the skills are substantially similar in the amount of education and training. In the Equal Pay Act cases cited by the nurses, the jobs were so similar as to be interchangeable, and where different skills are required the employer may explain and justify an apparent illegal wage disparity by showing that persons possessing the requisite skills are commanding higher wage rates in the local market.

In *EEOC v. Mercy Hospital,* (CA-7, 1983) 32 FEP Cases 991, the Seventh Circuit Court of Appeals held that the record supported the lower court's findings that a hospital's predominately male heavy cleaner jobs require physical exertion and degree of mental alertness not required of exclusively female and lower paid light housekeeping jobs and that the two categories of jobs are not substantially equal for purposes of the Equal Pay Act. It further held that the degree of the wage differential cannot itself serve as the basis for finding a violation of the act.

However, although it is not a comparable worth case, the case of *Brennan v. Prince William Hospital Corporation,* 503 F.2d 282, (CA-4, 1974) should be reviewed as the court held that where the availability of women at lower wages than men is the only discernible reason for wage differential as regards substantially equal jobs, such differential is prohibited by the Equal Pay Act as sex based. The 4th Circuit's decision in *Prince William Hospital Corporation* can be distinguished from the 7th Circuit's decision in *Mercy Hospital* on the grounds that the jobs in Mercy Hospital were not substantially equal for Equal Pay Act purposes.

In recent times, most hospitals have realized that they cannot have substantially similar job descriptions for both orderlies and aides (or other similar titles) with a wage disparity based on sex. Administrators should examine the job content of all jobs to be sure that employees are equitably compensated in comparison to others. It is relatively easy to examine skill, effort, responsibility, and working conditions for various jobs; adjustments can then be made so that job content is commensurate with pay and other forms of compensation. Job descriptions should be carefully integrated with the performance appraisal tool (see Chapter 9). Administrators who voluntarily work now to make their salaries more equitable can avoid the disaster that occurs when this issue is made into a union campaign issue or when equity is demanded at the bargaining table.

Two other court cases that applied the doctrine of comparable worth should be noted. They are:

- *Taylor v. Charley Bros. Co.* (D.C. Pa. 1981), 25 FEP Cases 602, where the district court ruled that an employer's decision to pay less to women in an exclusively female department than was paid to men who performed comparable, but not identical work in another department violated the principles of Title VII. In *Taylor,* the court endorsed the comparable worth theory explaining that, while the jobs performed by men and women in that case were not substantially equal, they were "characteristic of laborers work (in general) requiring little skill, education, or experience." The employees in the *Taylor* case all worked in a warehouse. All of the employees that worked in the repack/health aids department were female and were paid considerably less than the employees who worked in the exclusively male, "dry grocery" department. The court upheld the female employees' suit brought under Title VII and found that their lower salary was based solely on sex discrimination and that the discrimination was evidenced by the employer's long-standing policy of placing women solely in the one department where they performed substantially equal jobs for substantially lower wages.
- *AFSCME v. State of Washington* (D.C. Wash. 1983), 32 FEP Cases 1577, where the district court held that the State of Washington violated Title VII's ban on sex discrimination in compensation, as there was evidence of past discrimination against women manifested by direct, overt, and institutionalized discrimination that continued after Title VII became applicable and there was no legitimate overriding business consideration presented by the state.

Rounding out the comparable worth topic, the City of San Jose, California, authorized a job evaluation study performed by a management consulting firm which study highlighted pay inequities between male and female employees. The result was that the city agreed to pay a two to twelve percent increase for women workers, bringing the total increase to $1.3 million. And the State of Connecticut agreed, in negotiations with the National Union of Hospital and Health Care Employees, District 1199, to put one percent of the 6,700 health care employees' payroll, or $900,000, in a fund to remedy pay inequities between male and female employees.

In summary, the experts in problems of comparable worth and sex discrimination state that the marketplace economic principle of supply and demand should be the tool to close the wage gap. If it is not, the problem cannot be corrected without major societal disruption for courts to compare the hundreds of thousands of jobs with jobs of entirely different skills to determine if those jobs have the same intrinsic worth or comparable worth to the hospital. Many officials are unsure of the correct approach to the problem, since it is a major concern not only in private industry, but also in the federal government.

OCCUPATIONAL SAFETY AND HEALTH ACT

The Williams-Steiger Occupational Safety and Health Act of 1970 provides job safety and health protection for workers through the promotion of safe, healthful working conditions throughout the United States. Under this act, each employer must provide a work environment free of recognized hazards to the employees. The employer must also comply with the occupational and health standards issued under the act. Employees must comply with the rules, regulations, and orders issued under the act that are applicable to their actions and conduct on the job.

The Occupational Safety and Health Administration (OSHA) of the Department of Labor is responsible for administering the act, issuing standards, and conducting on-site inspections to ensure compliance with the act. The OSHA requires a representative of the employer and a representative of the employees to accompany the inspector during the on-site investigation. If no employee representative is available, the inspector consults with a number of employees who are familiar with the working conditions in the work place.

Employees or their representatives have the right to file a complaint with the nearest OSHA office and request an inspection when they believe that conditions in the work place are unsafe or unhealthful. OSHA does not disclose the names of employees who file such a request. The act further stipulates that employees may not be discriminated against or discharged for exercising their rights under the act; if an employee believes that he or she has suffered discrimination for this reason, a complaint may be filed at the nearest OSHA office within thirty days.

If a violation of the Occupational Safety and Health Act is found at an inspection, the employer receives a citation stating a time frame in which the violation must be corrected. The citation must be prominently displayed at or near the point of violation for three days or until the violation is corrected, whichever is longer. Monetary fines are also imposed when violations are found. Criminal penalties may be assessed when willful violations result in the death of an employee. Along with the mandatory provisions, the act provides for voluntary efforts on the part of both labor and management to correct hazards in the work place.

What To Do When the OSHA Inspector Arrives

An employer has a number of decisions to make when an OSHA inspection is imminent.

In *Marshall v. Barlow's Inc.*, 436 U.S. 307 (1978), the Supreme Court found that an employer has the constitutional right to demand a search warrant premised on probable cause. One advantage of a judicially approved warrant is shown by the case of *Weyerhauser v. Marshall*, 496 F.Supp. 1178 (N.D. Ga. 1980), upholding the necessity for convincing a neutral judicial official of the basis for inspection, thereby decreasing the opportunity for inspections designed for harassment. Also, a warrant limits the scope of the OSHA inspection as litigated in *Marshall v. North America Car Co.*, 626 F.2d 320 (3rd Cir. 1981). Further, the warrant works as a legal record to document the incidence and nature of inspections. Finally, the warrant provides the employer with some protection against petty complaints of labor organizations, competitors, and unhappy employees and ex-employees as established in *Marshall v. Horn Seed Company, Inc.*, 647 F.2d 96 (10th Cir. 1981).

The employer is entitled to be informed of the type of inspection planned. The two most serious types of inspections are those held to inspect *imminent danger* or a *fatality/catastrophe*. In these cases, the reason for the inspection is self-evident and a warrant is not necessary. The employer, however, will want an attorney present during the entire inspection, since violations cited by OSHA may also be used to adversely affect the employer in subsequent civil lawsuits.

If the inspection is a *general schedule* inspection, the employer has the right to know: (1) the criteria of selecting this health care agency for inspection; (2) if other higher accident-illness area employers have already been inspected; and, (3) that no other higher priority inspections remain at this time. When satisfactory answers are not forthcoming, OSHA should be required to obtain a search warrant (*Reynolds Metals Co. v. Secretary of Labor*, 442 F.Supp. 195 [W.D. Va. 1977]; *Marshall v. Weyerhauser*, 456 F.Supp. 474 [D. N.J. 1978]).

When the complaint gives rise to the inspection, the OSHA official must provide a written complaint to the employer. A warrant should be requested if this complaint inspection is not premised on the Occupational Safety and Health Act (i.e. that the written request with specific allegations about the nature and location of said problem was initiated by a current employee).

When inspections occur, be certain to limit the actual area inspected to previously cited items in the follow-up inspection or only items in the infringements cited. (See *Marshall v. Pool Offshore Co.*, 467 F.Supp. 978 (W.D. La. 1979) where the court limits the scope of investigation even in a general schedule inspection.)

The employer also has the right to have the scope of an inspection defined prior to the event. Even though a search warrant is the only way that an employer may be assured of limiting the inspection's scope, some employers are wary of insisting that OSHA obtain a search warrant. However, *Walter H. Kessler Co., Inc.*, CCH OSHD ¶ 23,415 (1979), was a case wherein it was established that an employer cannot be penalized for demanding a warrant. When a warrant is requested, the employer should ask for a hearing to learn more about the focus of the OSHA inspection and to verbalize any appropriate limitations in the scope of the inspection.

Conversely, if OSHA has a warrant, the employer should not allow an inspection to proceed if there is any doubt about the warrant's legal sufficiency. Contesting the warrant *after* the inspection means that objections must be heard by the Occupational Safety and Health Review Commission rather than the appropriate district court. It is to the employer's advantage to retain the right for a hearing in district court, rather than waiving this right by allowing the inspection to go forth on a defective warrant (*Southern Indiana Gas and Electric Company,* CCH OSHD ¶ 15,238 [1972].

In defending one's right to contest a warrant, the defense must be related to excessive breadth of scope or lack of probable cause to legally justify the warrant. The failure to successfully argue these defenses causes the employer to be open to contempt proceedings. Whenever an employer is served with a warrant, legal counsel for the employer should go to the magistrate's office to study the application and supporting affidavit to determine that all conditions are met for issuance of the warrant. Such conditions include the problem, the location and circumstances of the problem, inspection scope, time and day of the inspection, number and dates of previous inspections, specific documents that will be examined, and the existence of any higher priority inspections pending.

When the inspection occurs, the employer can be in the best legal position by proceeding as follows:

1. Realize that all conversations between the OSHA compliance officer and managers can be utilized against the health care agency.
2. The OSHA official should be required to meet in conference with management, prior to the actual inspection, and to present his/her credentials and delineate the purpose and scope of the inspection. This is the time when any trade secrets related to the investigation are explored.
3. When employers are unionized, the union representative accompanies the inspection party.
4. Answers to the OSHA official's questions on whether the health care agency is a business affecting commerce and under the jurisdiction of the act can be used to prove the OSHA case in any subsequent proceeding and therefore these questions should be answered accordingly.
5. Without a court order, the employer does not need to tell OSHA the number of employees in the hospital, as this information is utilized to calculate any penalties. Likewise, refusal to allow inspection of any records not covered by OSHA mandates and guidelines is prudent.
6. If the employer's accident/injury record for the past two years reveals a figure beneath the national average, the official must cease the inspection at that point.

7. The employer should accompany the inspector on the tour of problem areas identified in the warrant. Note all comments of the OSHA official. Refuse to explain, demonstrate, or volunteer any information.

8. With a court order, photographs or tests may be made. Note all testing methodology and tools. The employer should replicate any tests and/or take photographs independently.

9. The employer does not have to agree to private OSHA official-employee interviews without a court order. If the order exists, the employer may advise the employee that a hospital representative can be present in the interview upon employee request and that this time will not be compensated unless a hospital representative is present.

10. Do not pay an employee for time in an OSHA private interview where the employer is absent.

11. Avoid disclosing home phones and addresses of employees.

12. The inspection ends with a summary of violations found by the inspector. *Avoid* agreeing with findings or proposing a schedule for problem remediation, as these statements can be used against the hospital.

Contesting an OSHA citation that may or may not be founded in fact is a complex decision based on many factors such as (1) is the citation valid or has the hospital really violated the law and a hazard does exist; (2) did the hospital receive an unreasonable abatement period; and (3) what type of violation is cited; is it serious, nonserious, repeat, willful and knowing? A hospital faced with these choices should consult an attorney having specialized experience in the fine details of these cases.[11]

Unions are also worried about their vulnerability as a result of collective bargaining provisions that give them joint responsibility for work place safety and health practices, as well as work place exposure to hazardous conditions.[12] Employers may sue them for failing to exercise their duties under collective bargaining agreements. Employees may sue them for failing to perform a duty of inspection if an employee is injured. Employees may also sue unions for violating their duty of fair representation.

While employees have not won a great percentage of cases based on a union's failure to enforce contract provisions that involve employee health and safety, there is some indication that burden of proof is decreasing in some jurisdictions. In the state courts all that is necessary now to prove a violation is to show that the union has violated its duty of care when it does not adequately enforce safety and health provisions as set out in the contract or when it fails to warn employees about health hazards.

Unions are expected to respond to this trend in two ways. First, they will keep careful notes and suggest solutions to the labor-management safety committee so that they may minimize their joint liability. Second, contract language that now obligates unions to participate in health and safety activities will be softened to permissive terms. On the other hand, some aggressive union negotiators may take the opposite approach; they may take the lead in education, enforcement, and improvement of health and safety standards, with the hope of increasing their standing in the eyes of employees.[13]

To minimize liability, employers must make safety and health rules clear and enforce them consistently. They must heed the recommendations of the safety committee and risk management officer. They must thoroughly investigate any charge related to health and safety violations and obtain statements from all witnesses, since legal claims can be filed years later. In some of these suits, the employer may want to bring the union in as a co-defendant because of its duties on the health care safety committee.[14] Then an employee bringing suit must face the fact that the suit is being shared by co-workers and union members.

The OSHA caused a great stir when it proposed a change in the Medical Records Access Rule.[15] In late 1982, it was determined that the rule under Section 1910.20 would limit access of medical records to workers directly exposed to toxic substances. The streamlining of this proposal should have the effect of causing employers to monitor and keep records on work place exposures to health hazards. The OSHA intends to improve the detection, evaluation, and prevention of occupational disease under this standard. While this standard affects hospitals less than some industries, it posed a concern to all in regard to privacy as it was originally proposed.

In other developments, the OSHA is beginning an experimental program in which employers get a one-year exemption from general schedule inspections if they have a comprehensive consultation visit covering safety and health aspects of the work place. The OSHA is also involved in a nationwide effort to encourage voluntary safety and health programs. While such voluntary programs could result in freedom from scheduled OSHA visits, serious and fatal injuries resulting in employee complaints would be investigated.

Occupational Safety and Health Act Violations in Hospitals

The health care industry has more than 3 million employees in 7,000 hospitals and 1.7 million others in nursing homes and other health care facilities. There are many hazards to employees in hospitals, such as exposure to toxic drugs and chemicals, infection, noise, job stress, and radiation. According to records of the OSHA (even though hospital statistics are grossly underreported), 126,000 injuries and some 2,900 illnesses were reported in hospital employees during 1980.[16]

In January 1983, the *American Journal of Nursing* began a series of articles on hazards in hospitals. The first article focused on exposure to anesthetic gases and methylmethacrylate, a substance utilized to cement a surgically implanted prosthesis to bone.[17] Methylmethacrylate has been linked to a number of untoward outcomes in humans, although the incidence of such outcomes can be reduced by mixing the substance in a mixing stand connected to a ventilation system. Managers should read this series in order to become more aware of the health and safety hazards that currently exist in hospitals.

The Court of Appeals for the District of Columbia upheld the lower court that OSHA issue a notice of proposed rulemaking for a work-place ethylene oxide (a gaseous substance widely utilized in the health care industry to sterilize equipment) standard within 30 days and a final rule within a year to lower the permissible worker exposure level. (See *Public Citizen Health Research Group v. Auchter,* (C.A. D.C., 1983) DLR No. 52, A-6 E-1 March 16, 1983.) In the order, the three judge appeals panel stated there is "an obvious need, apparent to OSHA" for a standard that reflects the chemical's mutagenic and carcinogenic properties, and that the health care industry's efforts to protect workers have fallen far short in removing workers from the "grave danger zone." The court found that given these factors, it is "intolerable" that OSHA waited three years after the *Public Citizen* petition for an emergency rule to the projected final regulation.

The hospital laboratory is a place in which there are many hazards. Exposure to solvents, formaldehyde, mercury, and other chemicals can have adverse effects on humans. Chemicals of particular concern are freon, paracetic acids, ozone pesticides, and aromatic hydrocarbons. Toxic chemicals disposed of improperly can be a hazard to an even larger group than those in the laboratory. Contact dermatitis is also a common problem among laboratory workers, as it is among housekeeping employees.

Infertility, spontaneous abortion, birth defects, and mental retardation have been associated with exposure to hexachloride, neoplastic drugs, radiation, and mercury. Personnel can also have adverse effects from nuclear isotopes implanted in patients, microwave ovens, lasers, and germicidal and sun lamps.

The health of employees can also be threatened by hepatitis A and B, tuberculosis, cytomegalovirus, rubella, herpes, chickenpox, mononucleosis, gastrointestinal infections, and respiratory infections. Hospitals must encourage infection control by a qualified practitioner. A certification examination for nurse-practitioners in infection control will be available shortly.

Strict enforcement of policies dealing with the safety and protection of employees, the public, and the patients is essential. In-service education, both formal and informal, is an important part of the total health and safety program.

RELIGIOUS BELIEFS

Under Title VII, employers are required to take reasonable measures to accommodate an employee's religious beliefs and practices. The most common way the issue of religious discrimination could arise in a hospital is when an employee's religious beliefs will not allow him to work a hospital's neutral scheduling system (Friday evenings, Saturdays until sundown, or Sundays).

In *Murphy v. Edge Memorial Hospital,* 30 FEP Cases 1756 (U.S. D.C. M.D. Ala. 1982), the court held that Linda Murphy, a follower of the Worldwide Church of God, who refused to work Friday evenings and on Saturdays until sundown due to her religious beliefs, could be discharged where the hospital had a neutral scheduling system. According to the court the hospital was not required to alter that system to meet its Title VII requirements. Title VII does not require an accommodation where it would deprive another employee of the benefits of the neutral scheduling system. It also does not require the hospital to incur a greater than de minimis cost. The court found that it was impossible for the hospital to schedule the LPN to be off every Friday night without depriving other LPNs of their expected one full weekend in three and that substituting employees from within the existing staff would have required the payment of overtime, a higher wage, or decreased efficiency, thus entailing more than a de minimis cost.

Thus, if a hospital would not incur additional or more than de minimis costs by accommodating a certain amount of rescheduling, it should be very careful in denying such rescheduling to accommodate an employee who has a legitimate and sincere religious belief or practice. To avoid this problem, make sure in the hiring interview that the prospective employee agrees to work the various scheduling patterns that the hospital utilizes and also agrees to work required overtime and recognizes that working a variety of schedules and overtime work is a normal part of the job.

Finally, a court has held that a Connecticut statute providing that employees may not be required to work on their Sabbath has the effect of advancing religion in violation of the Constitution. (See Conn. Sup. Ct. 195 DLR: A-6, 1983.)

NOTES

1. "EEOC Chairman Thomas Says Comparable Worth Issue Hard to Address Because Law Unclear," *Daily Labor Report* A-10 (No. 191), October 1, 1982.

2. J. L. Finger and T. C. Greble, "The Impact of Age Discrimination Prohibitions on Reductions-in-Force," *The National Law Journal* 5 (August 1982): 18–20.

3. "The Employment-At-Will Issue," *Daily Labor Report* (No. 225), November 19, 1982.

4. Harold Hayes, *Realism in EEO* (New York: John Wiley, 1980).

5. John Forster, "The Dollars and Sense of an All RN Staff," *Nursing Administration Quarterly* 3 (Fall 1978): 41–47.

6. "Comparable Worth Issue Hard to Address," *Daily Labor Report.*

7. S. LaViolette, "Comparable Worth Rally Will Spur Lawsuits, Union Demands," *Modern Healthcare* 12 (January 1982): 56–58.

8. S. LaViolette, "Nurses Have 'Best' Case for Equal Pay" *Modern Healthcare* 12 (August 1982): 50–52.

9. Ann R. Miller, *Women, Work & Wages: Equal Pay for Jobs of Equal Value. Final Report to the EEOC* (Washington, DC: National Academy of Sciences, 1981).

10. R. J. Schonberger and H. W. Hennessey, "Is Equal Pay for Comparable Work Fair?" *Personnel Journal* (December 1981): 964–968.

11. Robert E. Rader, *The Employer's Rights under OSHA Law* (Ennis, Texas: McCarty, Wilson, Rader & Mash, Attorneys-at-Law, 1980).

12. Charles R. Goerth, "Employee Lawsuits Newest Target: Unions," *Occupational Health and Safety* 61 (February 1982): 35–37.

13. To receive an informative booklet on how one union is utilizing health problems on the job to advantage, write for *Hospital Workers: Who Cares About Your Health on the Job* from Public Employee Dept., AFL-CIO, 815 Sixteenth Street, N.W., Washington, DC 20006.

14. Goerth, "Employee Lawsuits Newest Target."

15. Deborah Schechter, "Medical Records: Who Shall See What, and When?" *Occupational Health and Safety* (July 1982): 23–26.

16. Jacquelyn Messite, Speech to 85th Annual Convention of the American Federation of Teachers, July 1982.

17. *American Journal of Nursing* 83 (January 1983).

Part III

Management Strategies Underlying Effective Labor Relations

Chapter 11

Improving the Organization: Effective Leadership Strategies

Since the beginning of time, people have been fascinated with the way leaders behave and the results they achieve. Leaders, whether formally or informally designated, share the power to influence others. Such power is derived from several sources, including position, personal wealth or "connections," personal qualities, expertise, and ability to reward or punish. Power, leader behavior, subordinate response, and acceptance are all inherent in the leadership process.

THEORETICAL PERSPECTIVES

In the 1940s and 1950s, those pursuing the formula that distinguishes leaders from others identified personal characteristics or traits. Research was focused on six basic areas. First, physical features, such as stature, age, and attractiveness, were studied, but there was no agreement about the ideal phenotype. Second, researchers focused on socioeconomic and educational attributes of families who created leaders, but they found a great deal of variability. Intelligence was explored as a leadership trait, but it was found to be only one factor among many. Other factors studied include personality, task-related characteristics, and social attributes. While leaders were generally found to have self-confidence, excellent interpersonal skills, a high task orientation, and high achievement and power needs, none of these were significant when viewed as isolated factors.[1]

In the decades of the 1950s and 1960s the importance of leadership style and effectiveness was emphasized. Major areas of concentration were the task orientation, i.e., priorities related to getting the job done, and employee orientation, i.e., affiliation patterns and concern for subordinates. Major studies during this time done by Ohio State University and the University of Michigan concluded that the mix of task and/or employee orientation in an individual's leadership style should vary in relation to the situation for successful results.

In the 1970s, studies in leadership were centered on leader style in relation to the total situation, including (a) the leader, (b) the subordinate, (c) the task, (d) the structure of the involved group, and (e) the type of reinforcement for effort. Two major theories were prominent, namely, Fiedler's contingency model[2] and House's path-goal theory.[3] Fiedler's contingency model emphasizes leadership style and situational favorableness, which is comprised of leader-member relationships, task structure, and positional power inherent in the leader's role. While the consideration of the factors described by Fiedler is helpful to practicing executives, House's path-goal theory is more useful because it takes into account four dimensions of leader behavioral characteristics. In House's model, the leader can analyze ways that decisions should be modified to suit the leadership style and situational favorableness. Because the path-goal model is one of the newest models, research findings on it are more limited. To date, criticisms center on its complexity and its limits in relation to performance.

As leaders continue to search for the best model on which to base their approaches to leadership, they should consider the reward power of the leader and the bidirectional nature of influence between a leader and a subordinate. In the decentralized setting leaders must also recognize the increasing autonomy that various units of the organization enjoy.[4–6]

If a hospital is to avoid unionization, its administrators must make a special commitment. Employees resort to a third party, a union, when management fails. An employee vote for the union is more often a vote against the administrators than a vote for the union. In order to succeed, administrators should:

1. recognize employees as their most significant resource and as important individuals (Exhibit 11–1)
2. implement a positive approach that meets employee needs so that the involvement of an outside third party, unionization, and collective bargaining are not necessary
3. bolster the confidence of employees
4. teach female nurses how issues of women's rights can be used against them[7]
5. learn from successful human resources management and Japanese management techniques[8]
6. temper traditional leadership and managerial duties with visibility, accessibility, and a healthy dose of humanism

Leadership vs. Management

Leadership is a transactional process in which an individual works to influence the goal-directed behavior of one or more other persons. Management tends to focus more on the systematic planning, developing, directing, organizing, and controlling of human and material resources required to progress toward the goals

Exhibit 11–1 Effective Leadership Is or What Do I Do Now That I'm a Supervisor?

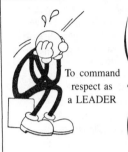

To command respect as a LEADER

1. Meet people, get along, orient new employees patiently, and encourage them to develop
2. Understand people and pick the right person for the job
3. Judge character, recognize potential, and use employee skills wisely
4. Communicate to people, think out and sell your decisions, and ensure that your employees know what is expected of them
5. Sympathize sincerely with employee problems, be sensitive to their needs, and tolerate differences
6. Motivate employees so that they work hard, put out high-quality work, and feel part of the team

of the organization. The literature is filled with discussions of the differences between leaders and managers.[9,10] Today's administrator needs to be both an innovator and a plodder who oversees the day-to-day routine of designing, delegating, and supervising the work that other people do. The required mix of management and leadership qualities is dependent on the individualized needs of each organization. An executive who succeeds nobly in one hospital may fail miserably in another. Fundamental differences in perspective between the leadership and management functions are highlighted in Table 11–1. Even when employees do not make these distinctions, they can readily distinguish the leaders from the managers in the organization.

ORGANIZATIONAL BEHAVIOR

Through the years, many models have been advocated as the "best" way to organize and administer the services of health care agencies. Classic management approaches tend to be rigid and authoritarian. Later models tend to be participative.

While participative models are largely successful, some complain that the prevalence of decision by committees makes it difficult to pinpoint accountability, expedite essential progress, and gain access to leaders. Others value the participative approach as one that:

1. bolsters trust and confidence between managers and employees
2. encourages positive attitudes, as well as intrinsic and extrinsic aspects of motivation

Table 11–1 Comparison of Leaders and Managers

Item	Leader	Manager
Preparation	Unknown, but often attributed to various combinations of personality, behavioral attributes, and acceptance of or power over and through others. No universal method of training	Defined tasks and procedures which can be taught through experience and formal courses in business management, economics, accounting, behavioral sciences, nursing science and administration
Focus	Change, innovation, creativity, commitment to push back frontiers	Order, continuity, routine maintenance, loyalty to organization and its mission, commitment to generating good will and tolerating circumstances that work to the benefit of all
Method	Scientific method with emphasis on inspiration and incorporation of new strategies into the system	Scientific method with emphasis on application of conservative ideas that will be readily accepted; consultation sought when tried and true methods fail
Goals	Doers who are active participants, who influence people to behave and think differently, altering what goals are selected as organizational objectives; goals are personal, even when they relate to the organization	Reactors who respond to goals as necessities of the organization, goals are impersonal and passively sought; good of the organization comes before personal preferences
Job security	High risk because of constant tendency to stir up novelty, change, and openness to new ideas; may move on when a new system is designed and implemented because of need for challenge and adventure	Low risk because of conservative approach and tendency to tolerate routine and pragmatic aspects of work, enjoys walking into a ready-made system that functions well

Table 11–1 continued

Item	Leader	Manager
Work	Artistic process of creation and synthesis that may occur in isolation; special style of influence to sell and excite others about the merits of proposed ideas; change or increased needs characterize work; ideas and work may be a mental obsession; may be difficult to separate the leader from the ideas	Process of mediating among people in and out of the organization to enable productivity, conserve and utilize resources effectively, and minimize emotional tension among participants in health care delivery services; attention to detail; coordination and balance are hallmarks of the workstyle; work product is communal, wherein the process and outcome belong to the organization; work is greater than any one person
Tool	Ability to influence others	Methods endorsed by system
Interpersonal relations	Concerned with ideas, empathy, intuitiveness, and the meaning of organizational events to participants; work sometimes done in isolation and sometimes with others; may seem disorganized, intense; people in organization stay in a state of flux and change; research and questioning attitude may result in interesting and innovative outcomes; predictability and sameness are low priority; power is needed to innovate and change policy	Operates according to game theory so that a win-win situation is reached; attracted by group and people activities; compromise and collaboration are major features of style; problem-solving methods often used; emotion minimized by the focus on how, why, what and when; empathy with individuals diminished by the emphasis on the mechanics of total operation; approach to interpersonal relations dictated by role played in the organization; often described as a "company" person who can be detached and manipulative; ultimate power and authority not essential

Table 11–1 continued

Item	Leader	Manager
Self-image	Belong to emotional forces and quests that drive them; life a series of goal-directed efforts, which, once attained, lose their capacity to motivate; struggle, change, and constant quests for change predominate; self-reliant, high achiever; one or more mentors often apparent	Belong to the organization, family, and friends; measure success by group popularity and ability to achieve and maintain balance; guidance of others and few stars in the crown; often satisfied to take a backseat to leaders

3. promotes a free-flowing communication process throughout the health care agency in all directions
4. results in open, extensive interaction patterns within and among all levels of the organization
5. disperses the decision making to all levels through group processes
6. emphasizes group input as an important value in goal setting
7. values self-control and problem solving as methods for controlling health care delivery and resource allocation and utilization
8. commits employees to high standards of performance by giving a high priority to their development, training, and management

The implementation of individual job and organizational designs can be difficult, however, since there can be so much diversity among organizations or even in the same organization over time.

In the 1980s, the continued growth in the number of health care agency corporations, coalitions, government regulations, and criteria for accreditation, coupled with more educated, involved consumers and more demanding employees, will influence the design and governance of health care organizations. Because the management style that prevails in an organization is the result of all these factors, plus the habits, experience, and personalities of individual managers, general management trends must be determined by each agency's unique situation.[11]

In nursing, the constant turmoil in which the nursing profession has been engaged has created great problems for nurse leaders who have been trying to articulate, communicate, and implement an acceptable pattern of management. Even through this period of rapid change, many nurse leaders have attempted to increase the ratio of professional to nonprofessional staff and have tried to progress toward holistic patient/family-centered care in which cost-effective primary care or smaller group care units are replacing large team assignment methods. Recently, directors of nursing have been included more often in the direct management of large health care agencies that have adopted a corporate structure.

There are no pat methods or models for managing nursing departments, hospitals, or other health care agencies successfully. However, management's quest for the perfect system has led to the study of organizational behavior, including:

- attitudes, behaviors, and performance of employees in the work environment
- informal and formal group structure as it affects worker performance
- environmental factors as they affect individual and organizational goal development, productivity, cost-effectiveness, quality of services delivered, risk management, employee and consumer satisfaction, and resource utilization
- employee attitude and performance as it affects or impacts on the productivity, resourcefulness, and operation of the organization as a successful business[12]

Key Characteristics of Organizational Behavior

The Contingency Approach

In the 1980s, management experts have focused on the interdisciplinary field study termed "organizational behavior." From research in organizational behavior, managers have learned that a realistic approach to agency management involves careful consideration of the individual, the group's personality (or syntality), and the organizational nature as the parts are interrelated at all levels.

Szalygi and Wallace present a readable, lengthy compilation of data on contemporary contingency styles. They emphasize the necessity of bringing together theory, knowledge of the organization and its members, and experience in a problem-solving format in which solutions are situationally bland. Managers who implement an effective employee relations program must first assess the opportunity for success by considering:

1. the individual characteristics, style, and power to operate effectively in the given situation
2. the followership as determined by syntality, expectancies, needs, motives, and past experiences of staff and administrators
3. the situation as evaluated through the structure and complexity of job tasks, the nature of leader-follower relations, the developmental stage of the department and the organization, and the expectations for group performance

4. the philosophy, power, and operational patterns of subordinates
5. the climate for executing the hospital's mission
6. a feedback system for continual assessment of productivity, satisfaction, motivation, turnover, and absenteeism in employees and consumer impact
7. a strategy for remaining competitive[13-18]

PLANNING, PROGRAMMING, AND BUDGETING SYSTEMS

The manager must have a system that maximizes institutional flexibility and responsiveness, staff respect and communication, and cost-effective programming within the limits of budgetary constraints. The advent of sophisticated technology; the rising inflation; the increasing official and informal accountability to the public, the staff, and the clients; and the need to justify costs for third party payers require a planned, participatory management approach.

Planning, programming, and budgeting approaches differ, but managers should commit themselves to some type of method that relates short-term action to long-range institutional goals and to a budgeting system. The master plan should clearly reflect budget development. Well-planned master plans incorporate all aspects of the staff, facilities, materials, and services required for patient care, research, teaching, and the public service inherent in each hospital. Alternative approaches to support the institutional mission should also be proposed. Concurrent financial planning should include resource acquisition, determination of priorities, and distribution.[19-22]

A budget is a summary of the institutional objectives, with their priorities, expressed in words, numbers, and dollars. The traditional incremental budget does little to evaluate goals, efficiency, or standards. Although a budget constructed along organizational lines to reflect expenditures is needed for actual operations of an institution, provisions should also be made in the budget to incorporate long-range planning in line with the institutional mission.

THE INSTITUTIONAL MISSION

Employees comply more fully with a program when the following six points are clearly delineated and communicated: (1) purpose, (2) philosophy, (3) objectives, (4) directions, (5) reasonable performance, and (6) resources.

Purpose

The most obvious purpose of a hospital and its nursing department is to provide high-quality patient care. A teaching hospital has an additional purpose, i.e., to foster a climate in which research and student instruction can thrive. Administrators must ensure that all departments within the hospital support the stated mission of the hospital. Furthermore, nursing directors must examine all their subprograms to ensure that they support the purpose of the nursing department, as well as that of the hospital. When the purpose of programs correlates well with the larger picture, it is easier to clarify the role of each department. The purpose has a decided impact on care at the unit level. For example, if an ambulatory care unit is to be a minimal care unit in which patients will receive very few hours of professional service, the cost of being housed there will be lower for both the patient and the hospital. If the ambulatory care unit is to be one in which patients practice their skills in returning to independence in activities of daily living, however, the unit will require professional nurses who are trained to help people return to their highest functional level.

The same line of thinking holds true in labor relations. When administrators make a commitment to employees as their most important asset, they must allocate the requisite resources. Too often, practice in personnel management is archaic "because we have always done it that way." In other words, the procedure or policy is one that is closely followed, but the purpose of such actions is unsound or unknown.[23]

Philosophy

While taking a look at the hospital mission, managers should update the statement of philosophy, which may have been written long ago. Instead of being a well-stated, but empty document as so many are, it should be succinct and helpful in explaining to employees the reason that the hospital values certain behaviors and strives for given objectives. In bringing the current statement of philosophy up-to-date, managers should ask themselves the following questions:

1. When was it written? By whom?
2. What relationship does it have to the realistic service philosophy in practice?
3. Does the document accurately reflect the main beliefs, values, constraints and current practice of the division?
4. Does the document indicate a realistic future direction for the division?
5. How does this document explain the relationship among the division and
   - the client and the client's family
   - the community or society
   - administration
   - nursing practice and other departments

- other health care professionals
- institutional commitments, e.g., religious, research, educational, charitable
- institutional administration

6. Does the philosophy coincide with a theory in practice?
7. Does the philosophy commit you to specific practice values, such as primary care, geriatrics, centralized education, decentralized administration?
8. What provisions does the philosophy make for conducting or applying research?
9. Does the philosophy indicate a commitment to a management style?
10. Does the philosophy explain the divisional/institutional position on labor relations and the employee complaint procedure?
11. How does your philosophy link the division to the appropriate profession at large?
12. Does your philosophy include collaboration, conjoint efforts, or cooperative pursuits with other health care agencies, education programs, or professional organizations?
13. Is there a statement in your philosophy that describes your cognitive approach toward clients, such as humanism, behaviorism, self-determination? If you utilize an eclectic approach, have you identified predominant beliefs?
14. Are client/human rights spelled out?
15. Are commitments to and rights of employees identified?
16. Are there more specific philosophies delineated for specialty units, such as intensive care, emergency services, psychiatry?[24]

The philosophy of a health care facility may fit into one of the following general categories:

1. operational. Often utilized by health maintenance organizations, the operational philosophy involves grouping patients in categories according to work required. Typical categories are acute care, minimal care, or patient education. In this arrangement, a patient is transferred to various areas to meet the needs of the workers. To those who advocate this system, the importance of cost-effectiveness and systems efficiency outweigh the problems incurred by the patients.
2. logistic. The philosophy based on logistics is popular, since it divides nursing care into parts. Such compartmentalization is familiar in many hospitals, since they have such units as orthopedics, neurology, and cardiac

care. This method does not allow patient grouping by acuity level or by human needs, however. While this method may cause some other problems in adaptation, such as the inability to move patients to balance the work more equitably among units, it is compatible with specialty trends and technological developments in health care.

3. holistic. A philosophy that has become a popular and important trend, the holistic philosophy focuses on the patient as a total person who is a part of many systems and subsystems. The patient's condition is described as a point on the wellness continuum and is viewed biopsychosocially in relation to the patient's total life space.

4. problem solving. In the problem-solving philosophy, managers use the scientific method to work systematically on all types of problems in the setting. As a result, many alternative methods and outcomes can be devised. Flexibility in fitting novel but workable ideas into the system is essential. The goal can be to maintain homeostasis in the system, whether that system is the individual patient, the employees, or the hospital as a whole.[25]

Objectives

In establishing annual and continuing objectives, the administrator should:

1. formulate measurable, behaviorally stated objectives that are congruent with institutional goals and resources
2. determine the amount of power or control needed to implement action toward objective attainment and assign responsibility
3. establish criteria by which to measure effectiveness
4. build in measures to ensure economy and efficiency
5. determine the role of other departments, clients, politicians, and other agencies
6. specify the equipment needed
7. determine the amount of physical plant changes needed to support the project
8. propose a budget
9. set specific deadlines for achievement of the objective in part or in toto

Only the implementation and evaluation processes remain. An objective related to labor relations is shown in Exhibit 11–2.

Directions

The activities or functions designed to attain an objective are categorized by Peter Drucker as result-producing activities, support activities, hygiene and house-

Exhibit 11–2 Sample Labor Relations Objective

Goal:	Improve management effectiveness in the nursing division of Your Hospital, USA.
Objective 1:	Practice effective labor relations. To accomplish this objective, the hospital will:

1. Educate nurse-managers through one all day workshop in labor relations and three minisessions of ninety minutes each during the next year. The workshop will be conducted in September, 19.., while the minisessions will be in January, March, and June. Each minisession will include a subject-appropriate film, while the-one day seminar will require Nurse Consultation Services to be hired as a conference leader. Mary Jones will be responsible for coordinating the education programs.
2. Identify and implement workable ways to reduce absenteeism by 50 percent by January 19.. One assistant director of nursing will be sent to a conference on absenteeism. The other five directors will be asked to poll their employees for suggestions by May of 19.., and to find a minimum of two articles in the literature on the subject. All suggestions and materials will be submitted to Tom Jones for analysis by June 15, 19.. A strategy meeting will be held on July 12, 198. and implementation of the plan will begin by August 1, 19.. Sue Zulch will be the chairperson of Project Absenteeism and will write a monthly status report on the project.

(*Note:* Fill in similar detail for the remaining subsections under this objective.)

3. Promote attributes of fairness, honesty, and consistency in dealing with employees.
4. Identify causes of employee satisfaction and dissatisfaction.
5. Establish specific ways to boost employee morale.
6. Assess and improve the method(s) for handling employee complaints.
7. Recognize the contribution that each staff member makes in a personal way.
8. Take an active interest in employee issues, interests, problems, talents, ambitions, and significant personal/professional events.
9. Show the employees that they are heard.
10. Seek employee input in all aspects of the management process. Communicate a commitment to participative management to employees.
11. Implement an open door policy.
12. Increase one-to-one and group managerial contact with employees.
13. Instill pride for and support of the hospital organization in employees.

keeping activities, and activities of top management.[26] As functions are identified and subdivided, they are delegated to areas, units, and committees for action. The further breakdown and implementation of organizational objectives continues with a discussion of job descriptions and assignment, staffing, and scheduling patterns.

Delegation is an order that must be accepted; it gives the employee the power to act and requires accountability. It is difficult to delegate work successfully and to manage human resources wisely, but the art of delegation is a necessary skill for the effective health care executive.[27] When delegating work, managers must ensure that directions are clear so that the involved personnel understand what is expected of them. It is unfair, obviously, for managers to give inadequate explanations and then blame employees for a communication deficit that is truly rooted in the delegation process. This managerial failure sometimes occurs because administrators do not know the frame of reference, background, and conversational level that is most appropriate for a given group of employees.

In order to delegate work successfully, managers must:

1. clarify goals
2. relate goals to the institutional mission and the current policies and procedures
3. define the job that each individual will be given
4. define the limits of authority and responsibility for each participant
5. set limits and deadlines for job completion in part or whole
6. open the lines of communication so that information passes over, bubbles up, and trickles down
7. institute controls

Managers who delegate work well:

1. are positive
2. know their subordinates well enough to capitalize on their talents
3. are receptive and open
4. tolerate error
5. delegate things that require a great deal of time, but little coordination and decision making
6. explain their expectations clearly and train involved employees thoroughly
7. choose the most cost- and energy-efficient person to do the job
8. record a calendar deadline for follow-up after the delegation action
9. *always* follow through
10. avoid taking a job back once it has been delegated, but are supportive and resourceful in helping the employee see the task through
11. give credit to others when it is due

Reasonable Performance

The requested behavior or performance must be consistent with employee values and role interpretation. It is unreasonable and maybe unlawful (e.g., in Florida) to discriminate against or punish an employee for refusing to participate in an abortion when the procedure is morally objectionable to the employee. Any requested behavior or performance must also be consistent with the organizational purpose and philosophy. For example, board members might object to a beer and card party in a Baptist Extended Care Facility, or they may disapprove a program on divorce if they are a Catholic hospital.

BOOSTING MORALE

To create and maintain high morale, low staff turnover, and effective employee relations, administrators must first learn what employees want from their jobs and then improve the work situation with this knowledge in general (Exhibit 11–3). Whatever the specific job-related changes that are needed, all managers can profit from following the Ten Commandments of Employee Relations (Exhibit 8–1).

Causes of Poor Morale

According to Webster, morale is the

1. Prevailing mood and spirit conducive to willing and dependable performance,
2. Steady self-control and courageous, determined conduct despite danger and privations,
3. Based upon a conviction of being right and on the way to success and upon faith in the cause or program and in the leadership.

When morale is low, employees complain of burnout and may exhibit lackluster efforts with decreased job interest, decreased productivity, and decreased quality in work output.

Causes of poor morale revolve around the lack of recognition and the failure to individualize approaches to various employee needs. In addition to working conditions that are inadequate or compensation that is inequitable by community standards, employees fault managers for failure in the human amenities and in the

Exhibit 11–3 Factors Important to Good Employee Morale

1. Team concept
2. Coaching and counsel
3. Opportunity to be heard
4. Consistent and fair discipline
5. No favoritism
6. Managers' sincere interest in employee problems and feelings
7. Loyalty
8. Credit given where due

people skills. Employees get upset when a trouble-maker, loafer, or chronic complainer is allowed to drag everyone else down. Hospital employees tire of "carrying" an employee who does not do a fair share of the work. They hate to feel that they are just warm bodies to fill slots. A popular journal recently featured an article in which it was stated that women have even more difficulty with institutional expectations than do men.[28]

Morale can also be deflated if employees feel that their complaints reach a dead end. Employees believe that they are entitled to be informed about the hospital's status and to have a voice in their own affairs. It is also damaging to morale when managers play favorites. No one likes to be given the worst assignment constantly. Sometimes it is not really the work that is so bothersome, but the feeling that a manager has deliberately been unfair. In other words, it is not *what* was done, but *how* it was done. Other factors affecting staff satisfaction and the quality of patient care:

- the need to provide hospital and nursing services twenty-four hours per day
- fluctuations in actual and effective census
- differentiations between direct and indirect care duties
- availability of supportive services
- working relationship among the nurses and between the nursing staff and physicians
- collective bargaining relationship
- time spent in nonnursing duties
- utilization strategies for assigning employees
- stability and flexibility of staff
- competence, expertise, and orientation of staff
- staff development program
- use of part-time personnel and floats; number and type of full-time equivalent staff members
- staffing patterns on all shifts, weekends, holidays, and vacations
- qualifications and job interpretations of leaders
- communication among personnel in and out of nursing
- physical layout of the hospital
- accessibility of the hospital to patients, suppliers, and outside resources, such as emergency backup
- absenteeism among staff
- status of physical facilities, supplies, equipment, and new technology
- philosophical and tangible support of nursing services by administration, the union, the board of directors, physicians, and community

- ability of nurse and nonnurse employees to understand patient needs
- changing patient care needs
- method of delivering care
- standard of patient care delivery services
- financial integrity of the hospital and adequacy of budgetary allocations for nursing services
- policies and procedures

Some Solutions

The people-to-people efforts to boost morale seem so self-evident that many managers simply take them for granted or fail to see the importance of little things. While the following list provides some beginning ideas for boosting morale, managers are challenged to take these suggestions only as the first of many others:

- Remain competent and in touch with areas supervised so that assignments and managerial plans are realistic.
- Compliment people who go the extra mile.
- Show warm human concern about employees as individuals by taking an interest in employee feelings, talents, ambitions, problems, and significant events in their lives. For example, comment on kudos that an employee's son got for athletics or grades. If the source of the information is the newspaper, clip out the article to give to the employee.
- Emphasize the importance of each individual to the total effectiveness of the team, in both verbal and nonverbal behaviors.
- Be honest and sincere in employee relations, being sure to honor your word.
- Be sensitive to the informal and formal hierarchy so that you may send messages through the grapevine.
- Be fair, forthright, reliable, friendly, firm, and consistent.
- Be creative in efforts to promote upward and downward communication.
- Show employees how their input is utilized in the management process.
- Strive to return all employees to the honeymoon feeling they had when they first started on the job.

In addition to the humanistic things that managers can do to improve morale, they should consider the anatomy of the job, the environment, the reward system, and the general interpersonal climate.[29,30]

IMPROVING PRODUCTIVITY

As a means of meeting the needs that employees express and of keeping productivity high, managers have gravitated toward the participative style of management. While participative management is not an end-all, it is proving to be a successful method for facilitating job satisfaction and productivity.[31]

Hospitalnomics

As cost constraints and budgetary curtailments have become the order of the day in hospital management, executive interest has shifted to an intense study of methods for increasing productivity. The first impulse of managers is to hasten to tell employees that they must conserve in every possible way. To many employees, however, such a mandate may seem simply one more order in an already over-whelming maze of orders and priorities. Employees respond in varying ways, but often challenge the administrator with a question such as "What good could my isolated efforts produce?" Because employees have their hearts in the aspects of their jobs that make a difference to them and to their clients, selling a program of hospitalnomics means persuading employees to commit themselves to the impor-tance of the effort expended both individually and collectively.

Patient Classification Systems

Staffing cannot be based entirely on the ratio of occupied beds to nursing staff on duty. The system of data collection, storage, and instantaneous retrieval must be developed so that nursing administrators may make realistic assignments of nurse-employees according to the level of care required by patients on each unit. This program depends on the hospital's computer capabilities and the development of a classification system through which patients can be categorized by identifying their need for nursing care. Staffing assignments may then be systematically based on patient care needs.[32-34]

To date, many patient classification systems have had limited use and effective-ness. Prototypic evaluation systems tend to rank patients by their degree of illness, but not all patients can be easily categorized by this ranking system. For example, a diabetic patient who is independent in hygienic and ambulatory functions requires extensive instruction during waking hours, but may sleep safely and continually through the night without requiring any nursing intervention. Likewise, care needs based on the degree of illness may become problematical when the acutely ill patient requires similar care on all shifts, since the most help is typically available on the day shift. Other patients may have fluctuating needs for care; for example, a patient who has a urinary tract infection may require the bedpan and hygienic care quite often until the medication decreases the sense of urgency. Still another problem in classification may arise when the patient is cared for by family or when patients with similar illnesses have varying capacities for self-help.

Task quantification systems are also associated with numerous pragmatic diffi-culties. To quantify tasks, studies typically utilize time and motion assessments.

Task accomplishment norms are established, and staffing is related to these norms. Historically, such studies were done by systems analysts who were not nurses. Adapted from mechanical industrial settings, task quantification systems captured only the observable activity of the nurse, leaving the psychosocial aspects and learning needs of care largely unquantified and, therefore, excluding a very significant aspect of professional nursing care from staffing recommendations. Task-related research also results in assignment of tasks to the most cost-effective person. For example, the nurse's aide is the obvious person to bathe a patient. If the bath needs to be utilized as a vehicle to assess the patient, to work on a psychosocial intervention, or to teach some aspect of home care, however the aide is not the correct employee to select for the job. Because nursing is a contingency-based profession, which observable activity may represent either the means or the end, task quantification may inaccurately represent the situation.[35]

Task quantification methods further ignore the fact that all patients requiring a given task do not have the same needs. Moreover, the nature of patient care is unlike that of work in factories, since the work situation in hospitals is subject to frequent, unpredictable changes. For example, a physician may do complicated procedures requiring nursing assistance as an unannounced aspect of routine rounds, a patient's condition can deteriorate into emergency status without warning, a visitor may have an extreme emotional reaction, or numerous unexpected admissions may arrive on the unit.

Task quantification methods based on isolation of tasks, task assignment to given worker levels, and homeostasis in the work environment result in unsatisfactory staffing. Quantification of tasks is useful in obtaining a rough estimate of work in a given area, but it may neglect the qualitative standard of care. Too often, norms in these studies are based on what *is* being done, rather than on what *should* be done. When discrepancies persist between the actual and optimal patient care situations, both patients and staff members may express dissatisfaction.

Administrators need a rational system for documenting cost-effective, quality service to their various consumers, accreditors, and health care providers. Progressive hospitals are installing a computerized nursing services scheduling system to facilitate communications among nursing, administration, and personnel, as well as to substantiate health care delivery costs. Such a cost justification system assists administrators in optimizing their use of staff, while giving the most efficient care. It also helps them to understand exactly what they are asking of their employees and what quality of care the employees can be expected to provide. Changes in reimbursement policies by Medicare and Medicaid rely heavily on the hospital's capacity to document patient needs in relation to services delivered.[36]

Cross-Training

Because of the increasing liability of hospitals for the actions of nurses who "float" to areas where they have not been properly oriented, hospitals develop the cross-training or sister unit concept. In this effort, specific guidelines should be designed and implemented, so that nurses are routinely and regularly utilized by other units that are similar to their primary unit of duty. Through this sister unit plan, staffing can be adjusted to equalize resources and utilize nursing staff more effectively. As a part of this effort, nurse-managers must analyze the daily, weekly, and monthly patterns of census and nursing care levels. Thus, staffing in each sister unit area may be made more flexible to cover fluctuations in staffing needs.[37]

Gaining Program Support

To personalize the effort to improve productivity, top managers may direct the following measures toward the nursing executive group:

1. orient the group to the present and future capabilities of the computer
2. update the group on concepts in productivity
3. break the group into smaller groups and assign each group an area of productivity to explore
4. ask each group to utilize education and other in-house resources to produce a twenty-minute presentation on the assigned topic with suggestions for realistic follow-up
5. have an intensive session with a representative group of leaders to ascertain methods for gaining commitment of the staff nurses to productivity-increasing efforts.

After the nursing executives have worked on this project for three weeks, each topic can be scheduled for presentation at consecutive weekly meetings. One group member should take notes for all group members, who will use them with the nursing staff.

To involve staff members in this effort, the nurse-managers should implement the sister unit concept. Staff nurses should also participate in the process of improving productivity. Their involvement may be requested by means of a letter calling on their professionalism to accomplish productivity-increasing efforts that can make a difference to them and to their clients. This personal letter on the "benefits" of productivity efforts should include meaningful statistics, such as:

- One unneeded registered nurse on a unit for eight hours costs $X per day.
- A sick call from someone who is taking a day off means . . . .
- It costs the hospital $X to grant each one of its employees one extra vacation day per year. If all of us can save $X, the hospital can provide all of us with . . .

The letter should also include a form and directions for collecting data about each employees's job.

The hospital may hold a contest in which the staff nurses are asked to submit suggestions on ways to improve productivity. Enthusiasm might be aroused by offering the nursing staff an in-service program that includes a short, lively presentation on productivity efforts and needs as they apply to nursing staff members on the job. At some predetermined deadline, the contest should be terminated. Suggestions that are implemented should be rewarded with a significant prize, money, or compensatory time, as well as publicity in the hospital newsletter. The public relations department may even wish to obtain community press coverage in order to show the public that the hospital is actively trying to conserve resources and save consumer money.

Evaluation

A mechanism should be established to assess the effectiveness of the program at each point. A personal evaluation form should be completed by everyone who participates in the effort to increase productivity. Statistics should be compiled on absenteeism, changes in staffing utilization patterns, requests for unpaid days off when the census is low, reductions in the uses of supplies, and other pertinent items. That information, coupled with the responses to the productivity analysis by participants, should lend itself to an effective study.

CHANGING MOTIVATIONS

In considering what today's employees can do in relation to what others did in years past, many questions need to be asked about changes both in employee characteristics and in the health care delivery system. What programs, benefits, or options must a hospital offer to appeal to contemporary employees? How much should management share the locus of control with employees? A shared voice in their affairs is as important to employees as it is to managers.[38] How can the productivity of current staff be increased? To answer this question, the manager must look at changing values in the 1980s in relation to work, quality of life, and expectations of employees.[39]

Instead of the Puritan work ethic in which work is the center of living and the main source of personal fulfillment, the desire for meaning in their work and the lure of increased quality leisure time motivate younger people. Although money is still a strong motivator, it may serve this function only until an individual's specific monetary goals are achieved. New motivators that have been recently popularized include flextime and quality of life programs.[40]

Flextime

First introduced to the United States in 1972, flextime has been heralded as one European solution to rush hour traffic congestion. Flextime (non-traditional work scheduling) is now being thoroughly explored in hospitals as a way to allow nurses to work fewer or more convenient hours.[41,42] Managers are concerned about this new option, however, because of the scheduling nightmare that can result from attempts to (1) maintain consistent levels of staff, (2) present acceptable work times to employees, and (3) contain costs by reducing overtime and maintaining the same number of personnel. Managers also worry about the supervision of staff members who come and go at odd times, awkward times of shift changes resulting in a possible breakdown in communications. Staff members who once worked as a group may lack the team spirit when they work odd hours with a variety of people. Not all employees like flextime. Once all these problems are tackled, employees may find that their initial enthusiasm for the system has dwindled with time.

Despite possible drawbacks, managers are making flextime work. Flextime has a number of advantages, including:

- easier child care arrangements and decreased costs for nurses whose child care-givers offer a daily rate
- reduced overtime through flexibility in covering busy hours.
- lowered absenteeism and tardiness, since workers can schedule their work for times and days more convenient to their life style
- increased leisure hours and multiple days off
- improved morale through employee personalization of scheduling

No one flextime schedule is right for every hospital. Hospitals should poll employees and managers to determine the most appropriate plan for each area. Baptist Hospital of Miami, Inc. makes these decisions by utilizing a task force.[43] Computers can be helpful in calculating coverage. Employees may bid for certain schedules with the understanding that they agree to remain on a given schedule for a certain time period. One option for scheduling combines two eight-hour shifts and two twelve-hour shifts per week.[44] Ferrel Hospital, a small rural hospital in Eldorado, Illinois, finds it best to have two separate staffs. The Monday through Friday staff works traditional shifts and receives benefits. The weekend staff works twelve-hour shifts, foregoes benefits, and is paid for forty hours.[45] Since flextime scheduling is becoming so prevalent, research is beginning to appear on the success of such plans.

Quality of Life Programs

Like businesses, hospitals are beginning to develop a wide variety of programs for employees or for the public with a special discount to employees.[46] Possibilities for hospital diversification include:

- a health spa with jogging track, racketball courts, exercise classes, sauna, and pool. This facility could feature programs and lectures on image building, stress control, time management, depression, and weight control,
- brown bag lunches with classes on all aspects of dieting and behavior modification. College credit may be given for such a course. Awards can be given to employees who succeed in reaching the appropriate weight.
- on-site college courses geared to the working hours of employees. Colleges, looking for ways to increase revenue, might jump at this opportunity.
- on-site child care centers featuring parent-child activities during the parent's meal time. Many hospitals are developing their own child care centers to attract employees on odd days and hours. Others are contracting with an existing facility to provide this service at reduced rates.
- lay courses such as Coping with Diabetes or Living with Your Aging Parent.
- a series of "fun" classes on many avocational interests that employees cannot usually pursue because of time constraints imposed by full-time employment. Group rates in special travel adventures may also be obtained by a hospital for employees.

In the quality of life effort, some hospitals offer employees the opportunity to take extra days off without pay when the census permits. Share-a-job and "mother's specials" work well for the employee who works during school hours and for the employer who must staff for daily peak periods.

STAFFING IN THE 1980s

Patient classification systems and cross-training programs have been discussed as ways of achieving appropriate staffing levels. Managers also must attain the appropriate staffing mix of licensed and nonlicensed personnel, however. In order to increase staffing flexibility for better balance in day-to-day practice, managers may consider ways of making part-time work more attractive and satisfying to nurses, or they may recruit a float pool of experienced nurses who have "stopped out" to raise families. Managers must take care not to make the float situation more attractive than full-time work, in which employees must work weekends and holidays. On the other hand, float staff might be more inclined to work if they receive some incentive above base pay and assurance that they will work only in areas where they have been cross-trained. In the search to make staff nursing a more attractive career option, hospitals have instituted *clinical ladders* programs, a system whereby staff can be promoted without leaving direct nursing care to become an administrator.[47-50]

UNDERSTANDING NURSE BELIEFS

Nursing has sought professional status for many years and the concept of nursing as a profession has been widely promoted in the literature. Administrators should refer to books such as *The New Nightingales* and *Nurse Power: Unions and the Law* to gain insight on contemporary thinking concerning union models for nursing. [51,52]

Many argue that there can be no professional nursing practice in hospitals, because nurses do not have authority over their practice in hospitals. [53] According to Kohnke, problems of practicing professional nursing in hospitals include (1) absence of professional practice models, (2) control of practice by the hospitals and physicians, (3) resistance to movement toward professionalism by other health care providers, (4) lack of staff and inappropriate utilization of existing staff, and (5) lack of clarity among nurses about what a professional nurse is and does. [54]

Role conflict develops when the professional becomes a salaried employee in a complex organization, as the individual has professional-client as well as employee-employer relationships and commitments. Some professionals have relinquished professional commitments to accommodate organizational demands. Others resist bureaucratic organization through resistance to rules, if performance is evaluated on rules rather than on outcomes. Blau recommended behaviorally stated outcome criteria as performance evaluation measures for a professional working in a bureaucratic organization. [55] Such performance appraisal methods have finally been seriously utilized on a widespread basis, [56] but the conflict between nurses as professionals and as workers in a bureaucracy has not been resolved. [57]

When work is mere conformity to rules, professionals cannot be held accountable for identifying proper goals and the means to achieve them; autonomy is a requisite feature in exercising control and in being held accountable. The rejection of bureaucratic standards has its basis in professional ideals learned in school, where bureaucracy and professionalism are viewed as opposites. However, the reality that patients have been placed in the hospital organization to receive the coordinated set of professional services that they require creates the problem of structuring an appropriate administrative network. [58,59]

The objective of professionals in hospitals is to gain access to the resources of the organization without being manipulated by the organization's goals of efficient coordination of diverse activities. Decentralization and the development of clinical ladders represent organizational attempts to accommodate nursing. However, there are still problems with the professional's universal service to humanity commitment and the hospital's value of material interests and profit production. [60] Because 65 percent of all nurses are employed by hospitals, nurses must find a realistic solution to the problems of being a professional within a bureaucratic structure. A balance must be struck between the use of peers and bureaucrats as guides in practice.

In a study by Corwin, it was shown that teachers resolved conflicts with less militancy when they became more professionalized. [61] In nursing, the American Nurses' Association has taken a public position as both a professional organization and a union. Such a position has resulted in increased militancy and has potential adverse consequences, as economics and strikes take priority over the "service ethic." According to Moore,[62,63] it is easy for a group seeking self-authentication of professional status to delude itself about the criteria of professionalism in relation to its group. Would the American Nurses' Association alter its current direction toward unionism if there were inconsistencies between its practice and its self-proclaimed norms? Can nursing educate enough capable leaders to promote the status of nursing within the health care system? Certainly, now is a good time to make some important moves to improve the status of nursing, because the entire health care delivery system is in flux.

NOTES

1. Ralph M. Stogdill, *Handbook of Leadership* (New York: Free Press, 1974).

2. Fred Fiedler, *A Theory of Leadership Effectiveness* (New York: McGraw-Hill, 1967).

3. Robert House "A Path-Goal Theory of Leader Effectiveness," *Administrative Science Quarterly* 16 (September 1971): 321–332.

4. Dianne E. Hendricks, "Opportunity for Managerial Growth," *Nursing Management* 13 (April 1982): 40–42.

5. Joyce Ross, "A Definition of Human Resources Management," *Personnel Journal* 60 (October 1981): 781–783.

6. Robert L. Trewatha and Gene M. Newport, *Management Functions and Behavior* (Dallas: Business Publications, 1976).

7. "Selected Materials Distributed at Conference on Organizing Women Workers," *Daily Labor Report*, Washington, D.C., BNA, January 29, 1981.

8. Richard Pascale and Anthony Athos, *The Art of Japanese Management* (New York: Warner Books, 1981).

9. Joyce C. Clifford, "Managerial Control versus Professional Autonomy: A Paradox," *Journal of Nursing Administration* 11 (September 1981): 19–21.

10. Peter F. Drucker, *Management: Tasks, Responsibilities, Practices* (New York: Harper & Row, 1973).

11. Henry L. Tosi and Stephen J. Carroll, *Management: Contingencies, Structure and Process* (Chicago: St. Clair Press, 1975).

12. Sidney Harman, "Worker Productivity: Technology or People?" *Personnel Journal* 58 (April 1979): 209–211, 253–254.

13. Kay M. Shearer, "Contingency Nursing," *Nursing Management* 13 (March 1982): 56–58.

14. Kenneth Blanchard and Spencer Johnson, *The One Minute Manager* (New York: William Morrow, 1982).

15. Hendricks, "Opportunity for Managerial Growth."

16. Ernest Jaski, and Marie Verre, "A Systems Approach to Increased Productivity," *Supervisor Nurse* 12 (April 1981): 29–32.

17. Thomas L. Kepler, "Mastering the People Skills," *Journal of Nursing Administration* 10 (November 1980): 15–20.

18. Andrew Szilagyi and Marc Wallace, *Organizational Behavior and Performance* (Santa Monica: Goodyear Publishing, 1980).

19. Drucker, *Management: Tasks, Responsibilities, Practices.*

20. Jeffrey P. Davidson "Communicating Company Objectives," *Personnel Journal* 60 (April 1981): 292–293.

21. Raymond McLeod, Jr., *Management Information Systems* (Chicago: Science Research Associates, 1979).

22. M.J. Riley, *Management Information Systems* (San Francisco: Holden-Day, 1981).

23. Drucker, *Management: Tasks, Responsibilities, Practices.*

24. Barbara Rutkowski, "Examining Your Philosophy," *Nursing Leadership: Challenges and Dilemmas* (Evansville, IN: Nurse Consultation Services, 1982), pp. 24–28.

25. Barbara Stevens, *The Nurse As Executive* (Rockville, MD: Aspen Systems Corporation, 1980).

26. Drucker, *Management: Tasks, Responsibilities, Practices.*

27. Patrick Montana and Deborah Nash. "Delegation: The Art of Managing," *Personnel Journal* 60 (October 1981) 784–787).

28. Natalie Gittelson, "Success and Love: Do I Have to Choose?" *McCalls,* November 1982, 110–113, 176–182.

29. Fortune Editors, *Working Smarter* (New York: Viking Press, 1982).

30. J. Ganong and L. Ganong, *Nursing Management,* 2d ed. (Rockville, MD: Aspen Systems Corporation, 1980).

31. Barbara Conway-Rutkowski, *Leadership: Challenges & Dilemmas* (Evansville, IN: Nurse Consultation Services, 1981).

32. Barbara Rutkowski, *PACE*.Information available from Nurse Consultation Services, 206 Charmwood Court, Evansville, IN 47715

33. John Forster, "The Dollars and Sense of an All RN Staff," *Nursing Administrative Quarterly* 3 (Fall 1978): 41–47.

34. Paul L. Grimaldi and Julie A. Micheletti, *Diagnosis Related Groups: A Practitioners Guide* (Chicago: Pluribus Press, 1983).

35. Forster, "Dollars and Sense."

36. Grimaldi and Micheletti, *Diagnosis Related Groups.*

37. R. Thorpe, "Cross-Training Program for Nurses: A Solution to a Staffing Problem," *The Journal for Nursing Leadership and Management* 11 (October 1980): 65–67.

38. Barbara Rutkowski, "Patient Compliance," *Nursing Clinics of North America* 17 (September 1982): 449–532.

39. Fortune Editors, *Working Smarter.*

40. M.E. Lange and D.B. Ardell, "Wellness Programs Attract New Markets for Hospitals," *Hospitals*55 (November 1981): 115–119.

41. M.S. Alivizatos, "A New Concept in Scheduling for Nurses," *Supervisor Nurse* 12 (February 1981): 20–22.

42. S.A. Coltrin and B.D. Bardense, "Is Your Organization a Good Candidate for Flexitime?" *Personnel Journal* 58 (September 1981): 712–715.

43. Roey Kirk, "Nurse Task Force Guides Flexible Scheduling Program," *Hospitals* 55 (August 1981): 60, 68.

44. Alivizatos, "A New Concept in Scheduling for Nurses."

45. Astrid G. Vik, and Ruth C. Mackay, "How Does the 12-Hour Shift Affect Patient Care?" *Journal of Nursing Administration* 12 (January 1982): 11–14.

46. Kirk, "Nurse Task Force."

47. C. Gassert, C. Holt, and K. Pope, "Building a Ladder," *American Journal of Nursing* 82 (October 1982): 1527–1531.

48. F. L. Huey, "Looking at Ladders," *American Journal of Nursing* 82 (October 1982): 1520–1526.

49. S.L. Knox, "A Clinical Advancement Program," *Journal of Nursing Administration* 7 (1980): 29–33.

50. E. Hines, "Career Advancement Programs: A Model to Identify Levels of Professional Practice," *Nursing Careers* 1 (1980): 4–6.

51. K.A. O'Rourke and S.R. Barton, *Nurse Power: Unions and the Law* (Bowie, MD: Robert J. Brady Co., 1981).

52. Patricia Sexton, *The New Nightingales* (New York: Enquiry Press, 1982).

53. M.F. Kohnke, *The Case for Consultation* (New York: John Wiley, 1978).

54. Ibid, p. 106.

55. P.M. Blau and R.A. Schoenherr, *The Structure of Organizations* (New York: Basic Books, 1971).

56. G.P. Latham and K.N. Wexley, *Increasing Productivity through Performance Appraisals* (Reading, MA: Addison-Wesley, 1980).

57. J.H. Ballantine, *The Sociology of Education* (Englewood Cliffs, NJ: Prentice-Hall, 1983).

58. R.G. Corwin, "The Professional Employee: A Study of Conflict in Nursing Roles," *The American Journal of Sociology* 66 (1961): 604–609.

59. Moore, *The Professions: Roles and Rules*.

60. H.M. Vollmer and D.L. Mills, *Professionalization* (Englewood Cliffs, NJ: Prentice-Hall, 1966).

61. Corwin, "The Professional Employee."

62. W.E. Moore, *The Professions: Roles and Rules* (New York: Russell Sage Foundation, 1970).

63. W. Kornhauser, *Scientists in Industry: Conflict and Accommodation.* (Berkeley, CA: University of California Press, 1962).

Chapter 12

Building a Supportive Climate

MANAGING CHANGE EFFECTIVELY

In today's world, change has become the rule rather than the exception. Coping with change effectively and creatively can mean the difference between high morale and productivity in employees and constant strife, conflict, and chaos. In order to manage the change process successfully, the manager must understand all aspects of change well enough to take an active role in directing it rather than simply a passive role in responding to it. When they can deliberately structure and activate the change process, administrators can move the hospital in a direction compatible with its mission, its objectives, and its employees.[1-5]

One helpful perspective on change is to view it in relation to systems theory. Every part of a hospital—employees, managers, board members, clients, third party payers, community members, politicians, physicians, or suppliers—affects other parts of the system. When directing change, managers need to anticipate the systemwide impact of change and plan the best way to return the hospital system to a state of equilibrium. Sometimes this means implementing a change; other times, it means resisting change in favor of a preferred operation already established.

In examining the merits of an idea, it can be helpful to apply the two-minute rule:

> Many executives' ideas wither on the vine for lack of expression to the right people, at the right time and in the right way. A quick rule of thumb for assessing your good ideas is the two minute rule.
>
> Next time you have an idea, clarify it to the point that it can be verbalized within two minutes. Such an idea summary should include the objective, why it is needed, how it will help, those involved, and any special costs in time, effort and money. Finally, include criteria for

knowing when your idea has resulted in goal attainment complete with target date deadlines. You will find it difficult to express "half baked" ideas this fully. However, once your idea is thoroughly focused, and you can express it simply in two minutes or less, you will find more people listening to you. Moreover, you will discover that your idea is ready to implement.

The two minute rule is useful in planning and communicating in all areas of management. Using the technique often is a great way to build skill in becoming more efficient and successful.[6]

In every hospital, some staff members favor certain changes, and others oppose them. In one hospital, for example, younger employees were pressing management for a child care facility that would be available every day on all shifts. Older employees resisted this, as such a benefit would not be useful to them. Management responded by creating a package of cafeteria style benefits from which employees could select a set dollar amount of benefits. This allowed workers with spousal health insurance to avoid duplicating an existing benefit by choosing dental insurance or the child care option, for example. When methodically promoted by management, this system created high morale and pride in the hospital's progressive policies.

Even when a change is a step in the right direction, managers should expect resistance. Employees like things the way they are. Change requires effort, learning, and adaptation; causes employees to wonder and worry about the outcomes; and threatens some employees. Managers must tell employees in advance of the change and be patient and supportive of employees while they undergo this uncomfortable process. Managers must:

1. think out and sell their decisions to employees
2. personally involve employees
3. maximize employee freedom while keeping control
4. identify sincerely with employees
5. train employees to succeed in their work
6. give deserved credit
7. hold employees accountable for assigned work
8. build respect and loyalty from employees
9. cultivate optimal working relationships by implementing the Golden Rule, being tactful, being honest, and being fair
10. recognize each employee as an individual and as a valuable member of the team
11. work to strengthen weak team members so that they do not doom the entire effort
12. emphasize the team spirit so that morale and group loyalty are high

Change is often characterized by three major phases.[7] The first phase, unfreezing, occurs when a situation arises that requires an approach different from any currently available in the hospital system. At this point, the hospital's disequilibrium becomes great enough that employees and managers perceive a need and recommend some change that would improve the system. The second stage, moving, occurs when people utilize the problem-solving process to implement change. The final stage, refreezing, is evident when the change is incorporated into the system and the system functions smoothly once again.

Change means difference. Because no two problems are the same, their solutions are not likely to be identical. However, most individuals who want to effect change can benefit by beginning with the problem-solving process:

1. Identify the need/problem/concern.
2. Obtain the authority to work on a solution.
3. Gather data and diagnose the problem thoroughly.
4. Define the problem by using the two-minute rule.
5. Eliminate unacceptable solutions.
6. Decide whether or not a change should be made.
7. If change is needed, devise the methodology for the chosen plan after assessing the feasibility, cost-effectiveness, and prudence of each alternative.
8. Identify terminal criteria of effectiveness.
9. Involve appropriate people in various aspects of the project.
10. Establish deadlines and controls.
11. Implement the plan.
12. Evaluate the outcomes.
13. Repeat the cycle in light of developments, as needed.

Problem-Solving Methods

Within the context of the problem-solving process, there are five basic methods that the manager may utilize, separately or together. With the *panoramic method,* the manager recognizes that there is no perfect way to solve a problem. Instead, the manager must select the best alternative after all options have been weighed. For example, a decision between promoting from within and seeking an outside person to fill a vacancy depends on the particular situation, including past practice.

Second, there is the *classification method,* in which the manager compares a current situation with others that have occurred in the past and asks what solutions have been successfully utilized for similar instances in the past. For example, if the manager is trying to improve communication with the chief administrator or the board, the manager might:

1. identify the current channels of communication
2. specify obstacles and facilitatory mechanisms
3. define exactly what is to be communicated
4. try to get the target person excited about the new ideas
5. decide whether credit for the communication or simple transmission of the message is more important, a critical point that often determines the success of the mission
6. keep the message alive so that it is not overlooked; send the message more than once in various forms
7. analyze the effectiveness of the approach for the future.

This method would also be quite successful in communicating effectively with employees.

Third, the manager may use the *critical factor method,* in which the manager finds the major obstacle and removes it. For example, one employee's pessimistic and negative attitude toward anything that management tries colors the response of those who work in the area. In order to identify and resolve this problem, the manager would ask the following four questions:

1. What is the most obvious problem on the unit? Usually, the most obvious problem is the major problem.
2. Have I honestly faced the problem? That is, can I set subjective feelings about a "sour" individual aside to assess the situation accurately?
3. How am I responsible for the problem?
4. What is the critical factor that will alter the problem and result in a solution?

Fourth, there is *innovation.* With this method, the manager strikes out in a new direction. Managers start to do this by attending university classes, going to workshops and seminars, talking to others at professional meetings, and reading and implementing what they have learned.

Fifth, there is *adaptation.* This is the most common method, because it requires managers to apply their unique knowledge and experience, both generally and situationally, to solve the problem at hand.

In applying the problem-solving process to preventive labor relations, it is important to realize that not every problem can be solved. The manager who cannot solve a problem immediately must work to minimize the damage it causes, however. Outside consultants can often add the objectivity that in-house managers may not have. Solutions that get to the heart of the matter often require time. Quick solutions are often little more than band-aid treatments, since they seldom allow enough time for employees to accept the change process.

Planning the Change

Prior to the initiation of a major change, management must be certain that the plan can be translated clearly to all levels of the organization. The plan should be defensible in terms of its present and future strategies, and it should be specific enough that top, middle, and line managers can determine their roles in relation to the big picture. Managers should also spend some time on consideration of potential problems or on simulation activities so that obstacles can be predicted and handled more effectively. Managers should formulate an explanation that makes employees feel a part of the change.

Once the commitment has been made to precipitate change, managers should ensure that employees are involved in every step of the plan. Management by surprises causes employees to feel negative and uncertain.[8] Before employees are involved in the change process, however, managers should consider how best to blend the values and talents of each employee with the institutional needs. As in the process of delegation, managers must clearly explain the performance they require of employees and what outcomes they expect. In addition, each employee should be told the degree of freedom granted to accomplish the assigned tasks.

Once the plan has been formulated and the guidelines stipulated, managers should build in an evaluation process that can be used both during the change process and at the termination of the project. Various types of evaluation at all stages of the project facilitate managers' ability to control and direct the change. Such evaluation strategies also allow managers to modify the plan, if necessary, in response to the realities of implementation. Evaluation techniques should be objective, as managers may be too involved with the project to be objective about its progress themselves.[9]

CHANGES IN LABOR RELATIONS

Tomorrow is a dangerous word in management. It is often the one word that gets managers into trouble with employees. When employees are disturbed by certain events in the work setting, they expect management to act. Many managers beg the question by reaffirming their intentions to solve the problem, but good intentions do not solve anything. Meantime, employees are experiencing mounting frustration and discontent. They want visible proof that management is trying to find a remedy for their problems, even if such efforts are not perfect solutions. When managers act to improve the work environment, they should share in the process with employees so that managers and employees can move forward jointly in making their hospital the best that it can be.

A manager caught up in the change process works in an assertive manner.[10] Assertiveness skills are applied as managers direct and control employees in the work relationship. Inherent in this process is the skill of persuasion. Managers successful at encouraging others to be cooperative are those who provide the facts, reasons, and explanations required, and answer all questions in a frank, forthright manner. They know the fine art of delegating and allowing designated individuals the right and pleasure of carrying out the assigned task, and they employ the highest ethical standards in all matters. To be persuasive over the long run, managers must remain reasonable in their expectations of employees, except in a real emergency. They must convey an empathy to employees. Persuasive managers are resourceful and persistent; they continue to approach important matters in a variety of ways so that the need for action is apparent to significant others. When they cannot keep their word, they supply employees with a prompt and satisfactory reason. Finally, persuasive managers have a special way of showing employees that they have great belief and faith in themselves and in those loyal employees who work hard in the organization.

POLITICS IN LABOR RELATIONS

Successful hospital managers are those who skillfully apply the principles of political science to their work.[11] Managers need skill not only in dealing with employees, but also in relating to peers, in developing those who are new to leadership positions, in relating to superiors, and in gaining support from political foes and allies tangential to the management process in the hospital. Some managers despair over the political nature of the management process, but they should realize that the practice of labor relations is political by its nature. The critical factor is for the hospital manager to understand the various relationships and sources of power, and to incorporate this knowledge into effective action on behalf of the employees, clients, and families who are a part of the institution.

Relating to Peers

Many supervisors in hospitals troubled with employee relations problems claim that they treat their own subordinates fairly, but that other supervisors do not. In many labor relations workshops, questions are commonly asked about how supervisors can cultivate trust, uniformity in discipline, and a spirit of cooperation in their agency. Answers are not easy. Many supervisors have good reason to be distrustful and critical of their peers in management, since there is usually a history of retaliation and negative experiences. Some settings are not appropriate for policies of enlightened management; one telltale clue to such a setting is a staff tendency to speak critically of "they," which can be defined as those senior executives who are scarcely visible to the average worker and manager.

In nursing, all managers should identify with each other so that, when someone in the organization speaks to a head nurse about what "they" in management are doing, that head nurse's first response is to affirm responsibility and authority for appropriate action in the situation. For the nurse-manager to respond in this manner, higher level managers must convey their support of reasonable interventions, their commitment both to the employees and to all levels of managers, and their feelings of cohesive group support. This requires frequent contact among all levels of managers, as matters of policy and business are continually relayed to front line managers.

Climate building is another important part of the process of promoting group cohesion and growth among managers. In order to represent management well to employees, managers need requisite skill training and positive communion with other managers. If the hospital management team is not really a team, it is necessary to work with caution, but also with determination, to alter the way things are. Each manager can assist peers and superiors in establishing esprit de corps in the group. [12,13]

If managers discipline employees in an inconsistent manner, a rotating board that convenes to review possible action in serious cases may be established. Such a board not only brings some objectivity to the situation, but also provides members with the opportunity to grow in their own management skills through sharing corrective strategies with others.

Some managers make the mistake of building good team rapport only in spurts. Managers need to be constantly reminded of the top executives' commitment to them in their difficult and often stressful roles as managers. Continual interaction and reinforcement is essential in creating a positive climate in which strong managers can work effectively with employees, the board, the community, and governmental and accrediting agencies in the people-intensive health care industry.

Developing New Managers

When polled about what they think will be the greatest obstacles to them in their new positions, new managers often mention the "things" that they cannot do. The important and most difficult aspects of management for the beginner, however, are the mastery and implementation of the "people skills."

An experienced manager should spend some time with each new manager in assessing the strengths, weaknesses, aspirations, and talents of the new manager. This may create a personalized orientation that combines the resources available in the hospital and those available in the professional community in a goal-directed manner. During this beginning breaking-in period the orientation coordinator and the new manager should specify deadlines at which they will assess growth and progress in the orientee's management skills. Such personalized goal setting should be integrated into the performance appraisal process so that such an apprentice manager may be recognized and rewarded for managerial growth. Likewise, the overseer of the process should be commended in the performance appraisal for effort in developing a new manager. Too many times, the effort of the learner and the trainer are overlooked in the system of rewards, which may be one reason that the indoctrination of new managers is not a high-priority function of seasoned managers.

There is no room for a sink or swim philosophy in orienting new managers. Poorly prepared new managers can be weak links in the organization, as they, too, represent management. Because they are "green," experienced employees may capitalize on their newness. Such actions add to the image of inconsistent, unfair management policies. From the perspective of the new manager, the feeling of being stranded may result in a sense of alienation and inappropriate identity with more senior members of the management team. Such outcomes only perpetuate the chain of making entry into the management circle disillusioning and negative.

Relating to Superordinates

Some managers are fortunate to have superordinates who are sensitive, progressive, and humanistic in their leadership roles. Others may not be so lucky. In the latter case, the only avenue to the implementation of manager's good idea may be to allow the superordinate to claim credit for it. Obviously, the utilization of the change process is important in implementing progressive strategies designed for the good of all of those involved in the organization. Managers should work both to support and to receive support from the superordinate as a necessary step in promoting the united front that is essential to the smooth functioning of the management team.

Gaining Support from Significant Others

Now is the time for managers to realize that the era of unending resources in hospitals and ever expanding programs has ended. Top administrators, business people on boards, and clients expect hospitals to operate as businesses do. Therefore, managers who expect an empathetic ear and a commitment in resources to their stated needs must translate those needs into language that business executives understand. An objective delivery of strategies and alternatives according to the problem-solving format is required to justify needs and subsequent institutional priorities and resource allocations.

Nurses must also become sophisticated in the politics and social skills inherent in business circles. As nurses close this gap with top administrators in hospitals, the entire management team is more likely to present a united image to employees. Currently, many hospital employees see a separation between top administrators and nurse-managers, and they may consider the latter rather powerless and ill-informed. This pattern is so prevalent that even nurse-managers may not identify themselves with the "they" in management. In other words, nurse-managers often relate to their employees as if they could not affect decisions of board members. Such role interpretation dilutes some of the effectiveness of the nurse-managers and perpetuates the large gap (sometimes called a gender gap) between the so-called top administrators and the rank-and-file employee.

Hospital administrators have themselves made some progress in closing this gap by promoting the chief nurse executive to the inner circle of top administration. This move allows them to receive direct input on the hospital employees who fall within the nursing division. Administrators must continue to build the skills of their top nursing leaders, however, so that these individuals can accurately present needs and information to appropriate support groups and superordinates, as well as to their staff members.

Luncheons, social functions, and fund-raising activities are an important part of reaching out to socially prominent community members, whose monetary and sociopolitical support is essential. In these hard economic times, wise administrators are learning to utilize some of the resources in the private sector to achieve the goals that traditional funding sources do not provide. Even if they are not involved in grant writing or fund acquisitions, all administrators should be informed enough to be good collectors of information that augments the resource acquisitions process. Nurse-managers can be good data collectors and staunch supporters of top administration when they understand that their efforts help to acquire resources necessary to fund desired programs and activities. Nurse-managers who can relate to all the various groups can be the best liaison of all among the various factions.

Hospital administrators who are not nurses have some of their greatest problems in relating to the work activities and needs not only of nurses, but also of other service departments in the hospital For this reason, they need to place a high priority on being visible and accessible to employees in all areas, even though they already feel pulled by board, community, professional groups, and political demands. Administrators who fail to convince employee groups that they truly understand work needs are in danger of having those employees organize, however. One comment that is commonly heard in hospitals where employees have considered unionization is, "We didn't get a union, but we sure had the attention of our top administrators for the first time. They wrote letters to us at home, met to hear our problems, and gave us salary increases that we never would have gotten otherwise. It's too bad that they don't do that all of the time."

HANDLING GROUPS EFFECTIVELY

In addition to relating to each individual employee, the manager must relate to the employees as a group in a way that facilitates goal attainment, meets both individual and group needs, and encourages interaction while minimizing conflict.[14]

Groups

Organizations are comprised of a number of formal groups involved in functional tasks and informal groups bound together by friendship or shared interests.

Whatever the type of group, the manager must assess its relationship to the goals of the organization. When groups are predicated on belief systems and missions different from those of the hospital, conflict, reduced productivity, and interpersonal discord may result. If such groups continue to thrive, they provide the perfect base for union organizing activities. [15-17]

Groups organized for a specific purpose, should be focused on task accomplishment and disbanded when the short-term project is complete. Different combinations of staff members should be rotated through groups so that permanent, cohesive bonds are not established. For example, many hospitals are attempting to improve employee relations and communication by having a randomly chosen, diverse group of employees meet for breakfast chats with top management. Such a group can be helpful, if management seriously considers group suggestions and implements appropriate action. When such a group remains together too long, however, they develop into a closely knit group. Such a group creates problems for management that far outweigh any advantages.

Groups form quite naturally among employees who work in the same area over a prolonged period of time. When management is attuned to the types of relationships that exist among these employees, efforts can be made to disband alliances by selected transfers of certain employees.

There are three main strategies that managers can use to modify the activities of a group. They may:

1. structure the group so its focus is task accomplishment
2. utilize the group as a part of the participative management concept, delegating tasks so that definite objectives, deadlines, individual assignments, and boundaries are agreed to by all (see Chapter 11).
3. redirect group attention to intergroup competition

Whatever the plan of management, the key is to plot a definite method of achieving the desired end products.

Intergroup Relationships

One of the more difficult aspects of being a manager in a large health care facility is in coordinating the various groups that must work together to utilize to the fullest the talents of all involved employees. Such intergroup coordination increases as the groups must interact and become interdependent on one another. The task becomes even more difficult when completion of a job requires a complex sequence of efforts from other individuals or groups. For example, the nurse caring for a patient with a large decubitus ulcer may require an order from an unavailable physician; a high-protein, pureed diet from the dietary department; special pressure-relieving equipment from another department; medication from the pharmacy; cooperation from the family; and assistance in moving the patient because the patient weighs 300 pounds. Conflict and frayed nerves may result when such a problem is only one of many that must be solved in a peak census day.

While meetings, task forces, and written policies are helpful in smoothing communications, they may not solve the overall problem. Some conflicts may be due not only to task performance, but also to power struggles. Departments within a hospital struggle continuously to increase their autonomy and extend their domain. Managers should strive to assist various departments in identifying and implementing cooperative strategies.[18,19]

Committees

In the movement toward participative management, hospitals have formed numerous committees to accomplish their work. Committees serve a useful purpose when their functions are understood and when they are appropriately utilized, but managers too often are so busy going from meeting to meeting that they have no time for personal contact with employees. Even though managers are doing great things in all those meetings, someone must communicate the progress to employees. Moreover, managers must take care not to use endless meetings as a way of dodging the human relations problems that are inevitable in labor-intensive hospitals. They should work to minimize the number of meetings held.

Committee Organization

Four basic types of committees are evident in most organizations: standing committees, task forces or design groups, groups based on organizational job standing, and interdivisional committees.

Standing Committees. Permanent committees established within the hospital and in each division are called standing committees. Typical examples include the patient care evaluation committee, the policies and procedures committee, the joint practice committee, and the new products committee. The types and functions of standing committees are determined by the institutional philosophy and mission.

Task Forces. Temporary committees created to investigate a designated problem and suggest appropriate solutions are called task forces. Members of a task force should be selected by their qualifications to search out the problem in question. Astute managers may also utilize the task force or design group to provide training for an employee who needs more information in the problem area. For example, the director of nursing finds that one twenty-year veteran supervisor has not stayed abreast of new developments in management. This is causing problems, even though the supervisor is well liked. To help the supervisor acquire the necessary knowledge, the director places this individual on a task force to investigate the feasibility of introducing a problem-oriented charting system. Under the cover of investigating the problem, the supervisor is updated.

Committees Based on Job Standing. Some committees are designed to include certain job designations. These committees should be structured to obtain the most diverse viewpoints possible on issues that are immediately relevant to the institution. For example, many hospitals have some type of executive meeting for head nurses, for the central senior executive group, and for department heads. Such groups should be formed only if they will serve a useful organizational purpose, however.

This type of committee provides a good opportunity for brief in-service training in expected role performance, as well as continuing education that is of value to practicing executives. Such an educational presentation can take as little as twenty minutes and may utilize a wide array of formats. For example, an administrator who decided that managers were not emphasizing the personal touch enough in their employee contacts may make a brief speech and then give the managers an assignment to meet with employees on all three shifts over the next month, to collect data on the feasibility of flextime in the hospital, and to report a summary of their findings at the next meeting. To avoid overwhelming the managers with too much additional work, qualified leaders may be assigned to assist them in the analysis of their findings in each area.

Interdivisional Committee. Another type of group that meets regularly in a hospital is the interdivisional committee. Pharmacy and Therapeutics committees are examples of such committees. The main purpose of this type of group is to reduce interdivisional strife while increasing communication. To avoid hard feelings, it may be helpful to rotate chairpersons. It may also be important to identify the power of the group to alter current policy; it is often best for such a group to be advisory so that their findings are taken to a higher level executive group for binding action. Because power plays are common in such a group, it is necessary to move slowly in pressing new ideas and to utilize less formal ways of operating. The informality allows members to become more comfortable with each other so that general relationships outside the meetings may be improved. Sometimes progress on agenda items of significance is painfully slow.

Ensuring Successful Committee Meetings

Successful committees fulfill several functions:

1. The group can be a status symbol—Use it to advantage!!
2. Meetings provide members with a sense of collective identity and a place where reality testing for appropriate limits can occur.

3. Meetings should help individuals clarify their roles, image and impact within the system.
4. Group decisions encourage collective support for ideas that are to be implemented.[20]

In forming committees, administrators must remember the following:

1. All members must know the purpose of the group and what is expected of them.
2. Carefully decide which groups should be temporary and which should be permanent committees.
3. The group size should allow optimal participation and functioning; that is, ideal groups have four to seven members. Ten is considered the maximum number.
4. Meetings need to be attended by members and skillfully directed by the leader to be effective.
5. The frequency of the meetings, and subsequent unity of the group, is determined by the tasks charged to the group.
6. The members and chairperson should be selected carefully to ensure group success.
7. If the task accomplishment is less significant than the improvement of politics and interpersonal relations, the chairperson should be skilled in achieving this end.
8. An ad hoc committee is a good place to accomplish the work of a large group, such as the head nurse group.[21]

Manager-Employee Meetings

Although manager-employee meetings can be difficult to conduct, they are important to every organization. There are two types of manager-employee meetings. First, there are the area meetings with the unit director that occur on a regular basis and often provide feedback on memoranda and meetings that have occurred since the last area meeting. Employees frequently voice complaints at this type of meeting if they feel free to speak without fear of recrimination.

The other type of meeting is one in which the director of the entire division or the administrator meets with all employees or small groups of employees. Meetings with the entire staff can be held infrequently when meetings between small groups of employees and the top administrators occur at least quarterly. It is often necessary for the divisional director to attend several meetings on each shift to be sure that all employees have attended. It is best if these meetings can be chiefly of the question-answer variety, although the chief executive may prepare some topics for discussion to start conversation flowing.

Staff members should be encouraged to offer suggestions or voice complaints. The executive should help the group clearly delineate the problems or issues expressed and try to provide any information that the staff needs on these items. When necessary, the executive should state that further research is required. It is important to follow up on issues raised at these meetings to show employees that their comments are seriously considered. Even if it is not possible to use their suggestion, employees should receive feedback to indicate that the item was considered. When the issue involves individuals, the situation should be equitably handled in a way that maintains individual privacy.

Informal meetings with small groups of staff may not occur regularly for two reasons. First, it is physically exhausting for the divisional director to work during the day and return to the hospital at night to meet with employees. The use of tape recordings or videocassettes to talk to employees between face-to-face meetings may be one helpful solution. Second, many top executives are intimidated by the threatening nature of such open interchanges with employees. In that case, courses and workshops are available to assist executives in leading groups, being assertive, and in handling conflict.[22,23]

A manager's motivation to come in at unusual hours, to exert extra effort, and to face employee groups is the realization that such efforts help to prevent labor relations problems. Organizations should reward such efforts both verbally and concretely through performance appraisals because they show an organizational commitment to the importance of each employee as the key to a smoothly operating, resource-efficient organization. Satisfied employees work harder and more efficiently than those who feel that management ignores them. Like lower level employees, managers need to know that their efforts are appreciated. The time and money spent to prevent labor relations problems are wisely invested.

CONDUCTING MEETINGS COMFORTABLY

When a manager conducts a meeting with employees, the manager must listen attentively. If recognition is deserved, the manager may tactfully give it to the deserving individual. If criticism is warranted, the manager must always give it in private.

The first step in conducting employee meetings more comfortably is to remember that their functions are to:

1. create a healthy work climate by improving employee attitudes and morale
2. improve administrative decisions by gathering input from involved staff members

3. promote team spirit among employees
4. present the management group in a positive light
5. discuss organizational objectives and philosophy in an attempt to improve insights into work planning
6. solve universal staff problems
7. promote staff development
8. share information and opinions
9. formulate more effective strategies
10. inform staff members of organizational progress
11. recognize outstanding achievements in employees and their families
12. ventilate feelings on current problems

Employees generally like to attend meetings with top management because they get feedback on the organization and can assess the impact of spoken information on other employees. Furthermore, the bidirectional flow of communication allows them to express and support others in verbalizing thoughts about the hospital and needed improvements. Meetings give employees an opportunity to assess the quality and sincerity of top management and to feel "in" on things. Not only do they obtain information related to job security, wages, and benefits, but also they get recognition for their loyalty to and productivity in the hospital. Above all, it is better for managers to provide employees with correct information than it is for employees to speak to less reliable sources or to an empathetic union organizer.

Meetings should start and end punctually. Meeting length depends on the topic, but no meeting should last longer than one hour because of problems in covering the work areas. Meetings on the same topics may be repeated in the early morning and late afternoon or on each shift to make them more convenient for employees. Votes taken at meetings offered at multiple times should be tallied for all groups before results are announced, however. Invited participants and the meeting leader change according to the topics addressed and the degree of centralization or decentralization in management.

An agenda can be distributed or posted on accessible bulletin boards so that employees can discuss the topics as a part of their meeting preparation. The agenda plans may even be shared with employees to gain the benefit of multiple suggestions as the preparations are made for the meeting. Meetings should be evaluated afterward with a representative group to improve the content and climate of future meetings.

The manager who is conducting a meeting should:

1. open the meeting in a firm manner
2. use humor wisely to break the ice
3. win group confidence by exhibiting sincerity, honesty, objectivity, openness, and evidence of preparedness

4. use audiovisual aids creatively
5. present problems in such a manner that employees sense the manager's personal identification with their needs
6. discuss current topics that are important to the group as a whole, stressing the significance of these issues by citing familiar examples and keeping the discussion productive and appropriate
7. get to the point quickly when the manager needs to present an item
8. explain changes thoroughly so that employees understand the rationale for them. A consultant may be invited as a guest when the manager's ideas need to be reinforced by an "expert."

In order to facilitate communication, the manager should:

1. restate a problem in a constructive manner to minimize group defensiveness
   - state the problem in terms of *what*—situation, activity, objective—not - *who*
   - practice sharing the problem with the group without injecting personal judgments
   - avoid opening discussion with a solution, with limited alternatives from which employees are to select, or with criticism of employee suggestions
2. clarify the problem, the area of freedom, and the task at hand briefly, turning the matter over to group discussion as quickly as possible
3. draw people out so that the maximum number participates
   - accept and reinforce member contributions positively
   - control disruptive members
   - acknowledge and encourage the expression of attitudes and opinions
   - protect group members who come under attack
   - recognize the inevitability of conflict as a part of group process and problem resolution
4. use pauses to advantage
   - allow people to think during pauses
   - wait long enough to allow different people to express themselves
   - break the silence by asking others to speak, or suggesting questions or ideas after a suitable period
5. expedite the meeting and the business at hand by learning to restate ideas succinctly, showing participants that the manager is listening to what they say
6. stimulate thought and discussion by raising provocative questions
   - encourage participants to speak and to share thoughts with small groups and with the total group

- avoid cross-examining those who voice comments
7. use good general technique to maximize the amount of business that is conducted
   - move discussion along by summarizing key points and indicating progress at appropriate intervals
   - restate the problem in light of current discussion
   - indicate differences in perspective among those who verbalize comments and seek further discussion on good compromises or alternatives
   - clarify group understanding, commitments, and responsibilities discussed so that postmeeting activity can accurately reflect meeting events

PREVENTING NEGATIVE ATTITUDES

One of the main purposes of meeting with employees collectively or individually is to prevent negative attitudes on the part of either the manager or the employee. An attitude is a

1. symptom of an individual's inner experience
2. response state derived from experience and personal reception
3. powerful factor that affects behavior

An attitude is a four-part process consisting of the stimulus, the affective response, the cognitive interpretation, and the behavior. A negative attitude can seriously impair an individual's judgment. Most commonly, negative attitudes are caused by (1) misinformation, (2) lack of information or training, (3) unclear performance expectations, or (4) stereotyping without adequate data. In the following example, Suzie lacks training, while the staff nurse has misinformation and unclear performance expectations of Suzie that result in stereotyping without adequate data.

> Suzie has been a nursing supervisor for ten years. A great deal of new equipment has become available in the period of time, but Suzie has not kept up with her bedside nursing skills. She feels out-of-date and marvels at the new responsibilities of today's staff nurse. She has not admitted this deficiency to anyone. In light of her problem, she has decided to stay clear of assisting patients who are attached to monitors and other complicated machinery. Therefore, Suzie walks past a cardiac patient's room to the nursing station when the call light is on, where she requests a staff nurse to answer the call light.

Which of the five categories has created the negative attitude in the above example?

1. Generalization. Staff nurse draws conclusions without sufficient data: she decided that Suzie probably felt "above" offering a patient a bedpan now that she is an administrator.
2. Situation. Staff nurse applies generalization to this specific situation: she silently decides that this supervisor is too "uppity."
3. Unknown factors. Factors unknown to the staff nurse: staff nurse does not know Suzie's reason for walking past the room. Staff nurse does not know that supervisor needs assistance in getting comfortable with new procedures. Staff nurse does not know the role that Suzi perceives herself to fill as a supervisor.
4. Conformity. Staff nurse decides to do what she has always done: staff nurse determines Suzie to be too aloof to know what nurses really think and need. She decides not to communicate.
5. Habit. Staff nurse believes that there is no reason to change the system or make waves: staff nurse answers the light, and berates the supervisor after she leaves the area.[24]

NOTES

1. R. Lippit et al., *The Dynamics of Planned Change* (New York: Harcourt, Brace, Jovanovich, 1958).
2. G. Zaltman and R. Duncan, *Strategies for Planned Change* (New York: John Wiley, 1977).
3. Amitai Etzioni, *A Comparative Analysis of Complex Organizations* (New York: Free Press, 1961).
4. D. Katz, and R.L. Kahn, *The Social Psychology of Organizations,* 2d ed. (New York: John Wiley, 1978).
5. W. Porter Lyman et al., *Behavior in Organizations*(New York: McGraw-Hill, 1975).
6. Barbara Rutkowski, *Nursing Leadership: Challenges and Dilemmas* (Evansville, IN: Nurse Consultation Services, 1982), p.8.
7. Kurt Lewin, "Group Decision and Social Change," in *Readings in Social Psychology,* ed. T. Newcomb, and E. Hartely (New York: Holt, Rinehart and Winston, 1947).
8. P. Hersey, and K. Blanchard, *Management of Organizational Behavior: Utilizing Human Resources,* 3d ed. (Englewood Cliffs, NJ: Prentice-Hall, 1977).
9. George Miller, "Management Guidelines: The Art of Planning," *Supervisory Management* 26 (May 1981): 24–31.
10. Malcolm E. Shaw, "Making Your Way Assertively," *Supervisory Management* 26 (March 1981): 2–28.
11. Linda H. Aiken, *Nursing in the 80's: Crises, Opportunities & Challenges* (Philadelphia: J. B. Lippincott, 1982).
12. B.L. Harragan, *Games Mother Never Taught You* (New York: Warner Books, 1978).
13. Thelma M. Lankford, "On Games People Play in Hospitals," *Nursing Management* 13 (October 1982): 73.

14. I.D. Steiner, *Group Process and Productivity* (New York: Academic Press, 1978).

15. Robert L. Kahn, *Organizational Stress: Studies in Role Conflict and Ambiguity* (New York: John Wiley, 1964).

16. Beatrice J. Kalisch, and Philip Kalisch, *Politics of Nursing* (Philadelphia: J. B. Lippincott, 1982).

17. Steiner, *Group Process and Productivity.*

18. M.N. Zald, *Power in Organizations* (Nashville: Vanderbilt University, 1970).

19. D.C. McClelland, *Power: The Inner Experience* (New York: John Wiley, 1975).

20. S.P. Robbins, *Managing Organizational Conflict: A Non-Traditional Approach* (Englewood Cliffs, NJ: Prentice-Hall, 1974).

21. Barbara Rutkowski, *Nursing Leadership: Challenges and Dilemmas* (Evansville, IN: Nurse Consultation Services, 1982).

22. Ibid.

23. A.C. Filley, *Interpersonal Conflict Resolution* (Glenview, IL: Scott, Foresman, 1975).

24. B. Rutkowski, *Nursing Leadership: Challenges and Dilemmas,* pp. 74–77.

Table of Cases

Index

About the Authors

BARBARA LANG RUTKOWSKI is the owner and director of Nurse Consultation Services, a business that specializes in helping nursing departments in labor relations, planning change, and in developing their leaders. She has been a faculty member at the University of Florida and the University of Evansville, and has spent seven years as an assistant director of nursing. Through the years, she has written extensively in the professional literature in her clinical specialty of neurology. Her *Neurological and Neurosurgical Nursing* text received the Book of the Year Award from the *American Journal of Nursing*. Dr. Rutkowski received her bachelor's and master's degrees from the University of Florida and her doctorate in higher education and administration from Indiana University.

ARTHUR D. RUTKOWSKI is a practicing labor attorney in Evansville, Indiana. He received his B.S. in management administration and his J.D. from Indiana University. Mr. Rutkowski currently serves as management co-chairman for the Interest Arbitration Committee of the American Bar Association, Labor Law Section on Labor Arbitration and Collective Bargaining Agreements. During his career, he has represented management in hundreds of election campaigns in combatting union organization. Since 1967, he has worked for both large and small firms in labor relations and orchestrating management programs for companies to remain non-union.

The Rutkowskis are the proud parents of three daughters, Laura, Michele, and Cheryl.